# Internal Fixation of
# Thoracic and Lumbar Spine Fractures

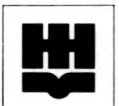

Walter Dick

# Internal Fixation of Thoracic and Lumbar Spine Fractures

Foreword by
Professor E. Morscher, M.D.

Translation by
James Wilson-MacDonald, M.D.

Hans Huber Publishers
Toronto · Lewiston N.Y. · Bern · Stuttgart

**Library of Congress Cataloging-in-Publication Data**

Dick, Walter, 1943 –
    Internal fixation of thoracic and lumbar spine
fractures.

    Translation of: Innere Fixation von Brust- und
Lendenwirbelfrakturen.
    Bibliography: p.
    1. Vertebrae, Thoracic – Fractures – Treatment.
2. Vertebrae, Lumbar – Fractures – Treatment. 3. Internal
fixation in fractures. I. Title.
RD768.D5313 1989        617'.151        87-26546
ISBN 0-920887-30-9


**Canadian Cataloguing in Publication Data**

Dick, Walter, 1943 –
    Internal fixation of thoracic and lumbar spine
fractures.

Translation of: Innere Fixation von Brust- und
Lendenwirbelfrakturen.
Bibliography: p.
ISBN 0-920887-30-9

1. Internal fixation in fractures. 2. Vertebrae,
Thoracic – Surgery. 3. Vertebrae, Lumbar – Surgery. I. Title.

RD533.D52 1989        617'.151        C87-094993-4


**German edition** published in 1984 (2nd ed. 1987)
by Hans Huber Publishers, Bern (Switzerland)
under the title «Innere Fixation von Brust- und
Lendenwirbelfrakturen», vol. 28 of Aktuelle Probleme
in Chirurgie und Orthopädie / ISBN 3-456-81616-2

ISBN 0-920887-30-9
Hans Huber Publishers
Toronto · Lewiston N. Y. · Bern · Stuttgart

ISBN 3-456-81624-3
Hans Huber Publishers
Bern · Stuttgart · Toronto · Lewiston N. Y.


Copyright © 1989 by Hans Huber Publishers
14 Bruce Park Ave.
Toronto, Ontario M4P 2S3

P. O. Box 51
Lewiston, N. Y. 14092

Printed in Germany

# Table of Contents

# Foreword

The goal of treating any injury is to restore anatomy and function of the injured part as completely as possible. Thanks to the advances in the field of osteosynthesis, we have come very much closer to achieving this objective in the treatment of limb fractures in the last quarter of a century. In contrast to this, a pronounced conservatism and even resignation has prevailed in spinal traumatology both with regard to treatment of neural injury and with regard to stabilization. «Well-established» treatment guidelines of pioneers in the field of paraplegia and lack of experience on the part of many orthopedic surgeons in the field of spinal surgery deterred many surgeons from making more intensive efforts to improve the changes of healing for patients with spinal injuries. Also the lack of versatile definitive stabilization systems for use in different types of fractures was a further impediment. However, the enormous improvement in the chance of survival for paraplegic and tetraplegic patients automatically provided an incentive to improve the results of treating spinal injuries, and enabled more rapid mobilization and rehabilitation.

The aim of spinal injury treatment is the restoration of spinal physiology, with relief of pain and restoration of stability without neurological damage. For many years, surgical measures were restricted to laminectomy, but this has become practically obsolete more recently because it is of little use and compromises the stability of the spine. Experience in recent years has clearly shown that the best method of decompression of neural structures is rapid and perfect reduction of the fracture or dislocation. Unstable injuries (however one defines these) are an indication for stabilization, or in other words for osteosynthesis.

The author of this work has analyzed the various current methods of treating injuries of the thoracic and lumbar spine practiced on patients with spinal injuries at the Orthopedic Division, University of Basle and the Swiss Paraplegia Center in Basle. In particular, he has described the weaknesses of the individual fixation systems. On the basis of his analysis, Dr. WALTER DICK has developed the «internal fixator». This was based mainly on the «external fixator» developed by Dr. F. MAGERL in St. Gallen. The internal fixator has various advantages over Harrington instrumentation which is used worldwide, not only in scoliosis, but also in vertebral fractures. These advantages are firstly the inclusion of only the affected motion segments in the fixation, and the ability to reduce dislocations and angulations much more effectively than with Harrington instrumentation. It can also be used after laminectomy, does not require many special instruments, and does not require additional external support postoperatively such as a corset or a plaster jacket thanks to the excellent fixation which can be obtained.

Transpedicular fixation of a vertebra, which was first performed by ROY-CAMILLE in Paris in 1963, has proved to be the most reliable method of fixation. Once this fact had been appreciated, the internal fixator became rapidly accepted in clinical practice. The publication of a second edition of «Internal fixation of thoracic and lumbar spinal fractures» by WALTER DICK and the development of a series of imitations of the original fixator are proof of this. Furthermore, it had already been shown at an early stage that the internal fixator was very suitable not only for stabilization of fractures, but for any type of «internal fixation» of the vertebral column. The second edition of this book has therefore not only been revised, but has also been supplemented by new sections which describe the applications of osteosynthesis in corrective surgery, in tumor surgery, in degenerative conditions, in spondylolisthesis, and other spinal conditions.

The fixation has been shown to be reliable in comparative experimental studies at the «Laboratory of Experimental Surgery» in DAVOS, and to date clinical experience has confirmed the laboratory results.

A further new chapter presents comprehensive followup results of surgery where the internal fixator has been used in 183 patients operated on at our own hospital up to October 1986. Thus the second edition is also a clinical audit, and documents the low incidence of

7

serious complications which occurred in application of the fixation.

Clinical management of spinal injuries requires profound knowledge of the pathology and pathophysiology of the spine. However, it also requires mastery of the techniques of internal fixation. Those individuals who fulfill these criteria will quickly learn to master with confidence the application of the «internal fixator». In our experience, this is the safest system for effective reduction of most thoracic and lumbar spinal fractures, and also provides long term and reliable stabilization. Furthermore, further indications for reduction and stabilization have developed in the field of orthopedic surgery. This book provides those confronted with the problems of reduction and stabilization of the spine with the fundamental knowledge they require, as well as a practical guide to application of the «internal fixator».

I would like to express my thanks to the Author of the book, my colleague for many years in our Orthopedic Department, and permanent orthopedic consultant at the Swiss Paraplegia Center in Basle, for his tireless efforts to improve the results of treatment for spinal injuries. I would also like to congratulate him on the development of an implant which has obviated many problems in spinal fixation which were not previously solved satisfactorily.

Basle, June 6th 1987          Prof. E. MORSCHER

# Surgical treatment of thoracic and lumbar spine fractures

## 1. Introduction

The aim of this work was to analyse the deficiencies present in the treatment of fractures of the thoracic and lumbar spine. As a result of this, a fixation system has been designed which is adapted to the biomechanics of vertebral fractures, and which is not a modification of a scoliosis correction system. In the second part of the work this fixation system, which is a type of «internal fixator», is presented. The mechanical design, the biomechanical function, and the experimental work are presented. Clinical experience to date at the Orthopedic Department, Basle University Medical School and at the Swiss Paraplegia Center in Basle is then presented.

### 1.1 Historical review

BERTHOLD ERNEST HADRA was a Silesian who subsequently emigrated to the United States. He was the first to fix a vertebral injury internally at the end of the last century. Prior to this, the only surgery had been excision of bone fragments or parts of the fractured vertebrae, which had healed either with pain or with compression of the spinal cord. In 1891, he stabilized a C6/7 fracture subluxation a year after injury. He used a silver wire tension band system, which he applied as multiple figures of eight around the spinous processes of the two cervical vertebrae [64]. He writes in his article:

«What do we do in other fractures, when the usual means de not suffice to keep the parts well adapted? We do the most natural thing in the world; we fix them to each other by direct means – clamps, nails, wires, sutures and so on. Now, there is no good reason why vertebral fractures should not enjoy similar advantages».

He pointed out that this procedure reduces and maintains the position of the vertebrae, and that it is applicable to all parts of the spine as long as there are no arch fractures, and that more than two spinous processes can be included.

This technique must also have been used subsequently by other surgeons in occasional cases;

FRITZ LANGE for example even used metal rod fixation of the spinous processes. ALBEE [3] and HIBBS [75] independently described the use of bone grafting for spinal instability in 1911 and demonstrated subsequent long term spinal stability. Naturally, these techniques were mostly used in the treatment of tuberculosis. However, laminectomy was much more widely used in the treatment of spinal instability at that time, and even L. GUTTMANN, who was later the most vehement critic of this procedure, recommended early laminectomy, presenting several cases in 1930 at the 6th Congress of the German Society of Trauma Medicine [63, 80]. With further experience, GUTTMANN discovered that simple laminectomy often gives rise to complications. In fracture treatment, laminectomy does not decompress the spinal cord or the cauda equina because the displacement of the vertebral bodies and not of the vertebral arches is the cause of the compression. Rather the original injury is rendered more unstable due to the additional loss of posterior bony stability. Consequently, GUTTMANN became a tireless advocate of non-operative treatment of closed spinal injury with paresis [62]. Subsequently, he improved greatly the non-operative treatment of paraplegics and tetraplegics by controlling potentially fatal complications, by postural reduction, immobilization in bed and rehabilitation. His revolutionary management of these cases led to the establishment of similar facilities throughout the world. Even today, treatment at most paraplegic centers is based on these principles [9, 50].

In the 1930's a heated discussion arose between MAGNUS and BÖHLER about the optimal method of conservative treatment of vertebral fractures without paresis. MAGNUS [121] proposed functional treatment ignoring spinal deformity, whereas BÖHLER [14] proposed closed reduction and restoration of normal bony anatomy by reclination and casting accompanied by early exercises. WATSON-JONES [202] wrote in 1940: «Perfect recovery is only possible if perfect reduction is insisted upon. Even a slight degree of wedging of the vertebra may cause persistent aching pain». NICOLL [144] advocated the opposite view, and showed that massive deformity in 166 miners did not lead to any impairment in the capacity to work, and that the lowest rate of symptoms was to be observed in patients *without* attempted repositioning of the vertebrae or surgical intervention.

The next developments in surgical management were proposed by BOSWORTH in 1942 [23], who introduced the H or prop graft fashioned rather as in joinery. More significantly, HOLDSWORTH and HARDY in 1953 [76] proposed internal fixation of the spine using double plates posteriorly which are fixed to each other on either side of the spinous processes. MEURIG WILLIAMS in 1963 [212] substantially improved the fixation when he introduced slit-hole plates with fluted washers. The stability of this fixation appeared to be so good that there was temptation to start early mobilization, and as a result there were numerous failures of the internal fixation associated with severe kyphosis. ROBERTS [159], in 1969, presented very disappointing follow-up results, but WILLIAMS himself had always insisted on three months bedrest following surgery. LEWIS and MCKIBBIN in 1974 [103] reported the late results of WILLIAMS patients, and although the results were better, there was frequently some loss of correction.

Hence fixation of the spine using plates to fix the spinous processes was abandoned. Even methyl-metacrylate re-inforced with wire or fibers has not improved spinous process fixation, and this is only occasionally used as a temporary measure [145, 146, 184, 203]. More commonly used nowadays are other more conventional systems, the most widespread of these being the Harrington system originally developed for the treatment of scoliosis. P. HARRINGTON in 1958 [59] first used this system for fracture stabilization. In 1965, WEISS modified the spring-loaded implant of GRUCA developed in 1956 [59, 60] to a «dynamic spring alloplasty» using it as a dorsal compression system for the treatment of fractures [205]. In 1963 ROY-CAMILLE started stabilizing the fractured spine with dorsal plates attached at the vertebral arches [165, 166], anchoring the system with screws passed through the pedicles into the vertebral bodies. In addition, he inserted screws

into the vertebral joints, thus gaining greater stability.

In 1977, MAGERL introduced the principle of external fixation for the treatment of vertebral fractures. Together with SCHLÄPFER, he developed an external frame [116, 117, 119, 173]. At the end of the 1970's JACOBS et al. [84, 85] developed a modification of the Harrington distraction rod, overcoming the weaknesses of this system in the treatment of fractures with improved stability, rotational fixation of the hooks and three plane adjustability of the fixation. In appropriate cases, anterior decompression of the thoracic and lumbar spine is used more and more frequently, allowing removal of posterior wall fragments, bone grafting and internal fixation [8, 18, 45, 91, 99, 129, 130, 137, 150, 199, 211, 218].

The controversy is still unresolved as to which techniques of surgery are best for injuries of the thoracic and lumbar spine, and there is still no consensus between surgical centers and rehabilitation centers as to whether surgery is indicated at all, and in which cases it should be used [9, 33, 34]. Currently, there is more consensus regarding lesions of the cervical spine since it has become evident that surgical stabilization allows early postoperative mobilization and rehabilitation. Unfixed bone grafts, as developed by CLOWARD [28] and ROBINSON [160, 161] for the treatment of osteoarthritis have been used in spinal trauma, but the grafts were found to be too unstable for fracture treatment [185]. Using special H-plates to stabilize the graft, dislocation of the graft could be avoided. The use of plates for anterior spinal fixation rapidly gained worldwide popularity in the 1970's encouraged by publications from OROZCO and LLOVET [147] as well as SENEGAS and GAUZERE [179], and has proved to be effective as a standard technique. Precursors of metal fixation using anterior bone grafts were described by SCHÜRMANN and BUSCH [177], JUNGHANNS [88], TSCHERNE [193, 194] as well as BÖHLER [13], but these have been outdated and replaced by simpler H-plates as well as interbody bone cement plugging [58, 151]. In 1982, CASPAR presented a plate with double slits for fixation of the cervical spine [26]. More recently, MORSCHER [133] has developed a titanium plate with hollow screws locking in the plate hole where bone growing into the hollow spaces within the screws improves stability.

## 1.2 Current surgical management of vertebral fractures

The indications for internal fixation of vertebral fractures are as yet undetermined, as was the case for fractures elsewhere in the skeleton two or three decades ago. However, for the rest of skeleton there is now more agreement about the different approaches to treatment. The delay in development of internal fixation of spinal fractures is due to the following causes:

- Because many different anatomical structures are affected by the injury, there is great diversity in the different types of spinal injury [135], and until now an adequate classification has not been available. Because of this, it is not possible to compare different patient groups adequately. In contrast, in the rest of the skeleton extensive documentation of types of injury has allowed comparison of individual methods of treatment. This difference is only gradually being corrected with the studies of DENIS [35] and MCAFEE [125, 126].
- The majority of vertebral fractures are simple compression fractures, and hence conservative management is usually appropriate, as in the majority of radial fractures. Thus only a few severe spinal injuries are collected by any particular clinician, which makes statistical comparison between different types of treatment almost impossible because of the small numbers.
- «Functional treatment», with early mobilization which is one of the main aims in the surgical treatment of fractures is possible in the majority of vertebral fractures, even when conservative treatment is used, and this has been practiced for decades.
- Another important principle of surgical treatment of fractures, namely restoration of joint congruity, is not possible in the treatment of vertebral fractures. Indeed, until now several healthy joints have often been included in the fixation or fusion, and in fixation of five or six motion segments, for example, significant morbidity may occur due to this, especially for a paraplegic patient.
- Requirement for «exercise stability» of the

osteosynthesis simultaneously demands «loading stability», to allow mobilization of the patient. The achievement of «positional stability» with internal fixation does not bring about any major advantage over conservative management, and merely adds together the risks of the two forms of treatment.

- The vertebral column is not only an organ allowing movement, but also carries the spinal cord. If the trauma causes a primary spinal cord injury, this is irreversible and is currently not treatable surgically. Only secondary functional deficits caused by spinal shock, edema, hematoma or spinal compression due to bone fragments within the canal can recover. If there is no primary cord injury compression due to fracture fragments can often be eliminated by closed reduction as well as by surgery. Thus surgical treatment of vertebral fractures where there is neurological damage must on the one hand eliminate any factors which might impair spontaneous recovery of reversible injury, and of course avoid the risk of additional damage. On the other hand, the main aim of surgery should be to allow early rehabilitation immediately after injury, as well as improving the subsequent life style of the patient. In the first era of surgical therapy, the only concern was to decompress the spinal cord, and treatment of the fracture and the biomechanical function of the spine were ignored. Laminectomy was widely used to achieve decompression of the spinal cord rather than for fracture repositioning or removal of anterior fragments, and this was clearly unsuitable. Additional instability was created, and it is now understood that laminectomy in these cases was doomed to failure.
- A dramatic fall in the mortality of individuals with spinal injuries of the cervical or thoracic spinal cord with paraplegia has occurred because of the prevention of secondary complications, and is largely independent of the type of treatment used for the fracture itself.
- Extensive spinal injury with paraplegia or tetraplegia requires highly specialized treatment centers because of the intensive nursing required. These have mostly been built remote from centers of acute medical treatment out in the country, which is understandable due to

the timing of their development. They do not have operating facilities and staff of their own, and are unable to build up such facilities because of the cost. Conversely, trauma services cannot assume responsibility for the entire treatment of this group of injured persons. However, for the development of surgical treatment, close collaboration of all disciplines involved is necessary, and such teams have only been forming in recent years.

In spite of the above difficulties, we are confronted by the need to put more emphasis on surgical treatment of spinal fractures in order to improve overall treatment. This is because conservative treatment, which has been perfected over more than 50 years , has reached its limits. Two prerequisites which make development of spinal surgery easier are firstly, that standard approaches are available which make any part of the spine accessible either posteriorly or anteriorly, and secondly, that new imaging techniques such as polytomography [5] and computerized tomography [21, 55, 104, 191, 210] have considerably improved our knowledge and three dimensional appreciation of spinal injuries. This information allows us to analyse the pathology of each individual case based on the biomechanics of the spine [10, 77, 78, 144, 158, 206, 208, 215]. In the near future, MRI will allow us to evaluate further injuries of the spinal cord itself.

However, it is necessary to specify two other prerequisites; these are first, to improve understanding of the indications for internal fixation based on clinical trials, and secondly, above all, to improve fixation systems which are designed from the start to stabilize the traumatized spine rather than to adapt scoliosis instrumentations, which are designed on the assumption that the ligaments and vertebral bodies are intact. The development of the plates of ROY-CAMILLE and the external fixator of MAGERL and SCHLÄPFER have already come some way towards achieving this; a new fracture stabilization system which works on the same principle as the external fixator, but which is implantable is to be presented in this paper.

## 2. Requirements of fixation

### 2.1 Vertebral fractures without neurological injury

Requirements of an internal fixation system of the spine are similar to those in general traumatology.

*a)* The material from which the implant is made must by biocompatible. This is not a problem since suitable implant materials are available.

*b)* In the surgical treatment of fractures, «exercise stability» is to be achieved which allows mobilization. In the limbs, this entails non-weight bearing active movement. However, the spine cannot be freed from the body weight cranial to the fracture, nor from the forces applied by the spinal musculature in the erect posture, which may be greater than the weight being carried. Hence, the implant must be able to absorb and neutralize these forces by its intrinsic stability and also by the stability of fixation to the skeleton. If adequate stability is not attained and a long period of confinement to bed or plaster splintage is necessary postoperatively, the risks of surgical infection and anesthesia are only added to the disadvantages of conservative treatment. The justification of surgical treatment is then questionable. At most, a light, three-point corset is acceptable.

However, reliable measurements of the forces and bending moments acting on the spine during life do not exist, and will not be obtainable in the forseeable future. Only in vivo measurements of the intravertebral disc pressure [139], axial pressure [139], axial pressure measurements on the Harrington rod in scoliosis corrections [140] and sagittal bending moments measured on an external fixator of the spine [172, 214] are known. With simplified assumptions about the weight of body segments and their center of gravity, the ventral bending moment can be estimated to be about 25 Nm in the erect posture with an increase to 80 Nm at 90° of forward flexion with muscle relaxation (WHITE and PANJABI [202] and JACOBS, NORDWALL and NACHEMSON [83]). WÖRSDÖRFER [214] measured an a.p. bending moment of only 8 Nm using an external fixator in 6 patients with vertebral fractures, and QUIN-

NELL et al. [154] measured very much lower intradiscal pressures than NACHEMSON [139].

At the moment, no definite minimum values can be calculated, and only clinical experience and observation will enable it to be decided which implants show the necessary stability, and which are their weak points. In the development of new implants, the relative stability of any one implant can of course be investigated experimentally by comparing with implants which have already been used clinically, so that any improvements in the implant can be measured and tested before being put to clinical use [214].

*c)* The implant should restore anatomy. In spinal trauma, this does not mean the repositioning of every individual small fragment, but the restoration of the basic shape of the affected spinal region in physiological lordosis or kyphosis, with the elimination of angular deformity and displacement of the main vertebral fragments.

*d)* The fixation system should ensure stability of the injured part of the vertebral column even when there are substantial bony defects or ligamentous injuries. The fixation should be designed biomechanically in such a way that it can be used as well when there is a complete ligamentous injury, a fractured posterior wall or a loss of bone stock in the vertebral body, since it is important to be able to fix internally very unstable spinal injuries by surgical means.

## 2.2 Vertebral fractures with neurological injury

In fractures of the thoracolumbar spine with paraplegia, there is a further requirement of the implant which is crucially important, and which also applies to fractures without neurological complications:

The paraplegic patient depends on extensive mobility of the lumbar spine for rehabilitation, and this will be dealt with in more detail later. The mobility of the uninjured segments must be preserved, and this means that the implant should not compromise more than the two adjacent vertebrae involved in the injury, and should only immobilize these.

## 3. Indications for surgical treatment

### 3.1 Vertebral fractures without neurological injury

Treatment of vertebral fractures and fracture dislocations should be carried out in accordance with the principles which apply to general fracture theory. These consist of repositioning where necessary, and maintenance of anatomy until bony healing occurs in such a way that satisfactory function can be expected. In the vast majority of cases of vertebral injury, treatment remains conservative. The indications for surgery are:

*a)* All dislocations and fracture dislocations, which are unreducible by closed means (Fig. 1).

*b)* Persistent unstable spinal injuries. These are the injuries which will almost certainly never become stable even *after* bony consolidation of the fracture (Fig. 2), because simultaneous rupture of the intervertebral disc and the dorsal capsular ligament complex constitutes the main part of the injury. In contrast to cancellous fractures, such ligamentous injuries only heal by scar formation which is too weak and lax.

*c)* Where there is a large defect in the vertebral body anteriorly, the deformity remaining after healing has occurred may lead to long term symptoms due to the resulting kyphosis. In practice, this is a great problem because it is difficult to predict whether the reduction will be maintained with good conservative treatment, or whether a secondary kyphosis will develop. Figures 3a and b illustrate these differences. However, it is difficult to predict what degree of kyphotic spinal deformity or compensatory lordosis will lead to pain in a specific patient, since the individual differences are very great. Many factors play a role in the development of pain, not least psychological factors, and also whether or not the patient is insured [105]. NICOLL [144] reports on very severe kyphotic deformities in working miners with few symptoms, but every clinician knows patients with only moderate kyphoses who complain of long standing pain induced by secondary degenerative changes in the intervertebral joints due to an abnormal posture, either in the kyphosis itself, or in the region of the compensatory lumbar hyperlordosis.

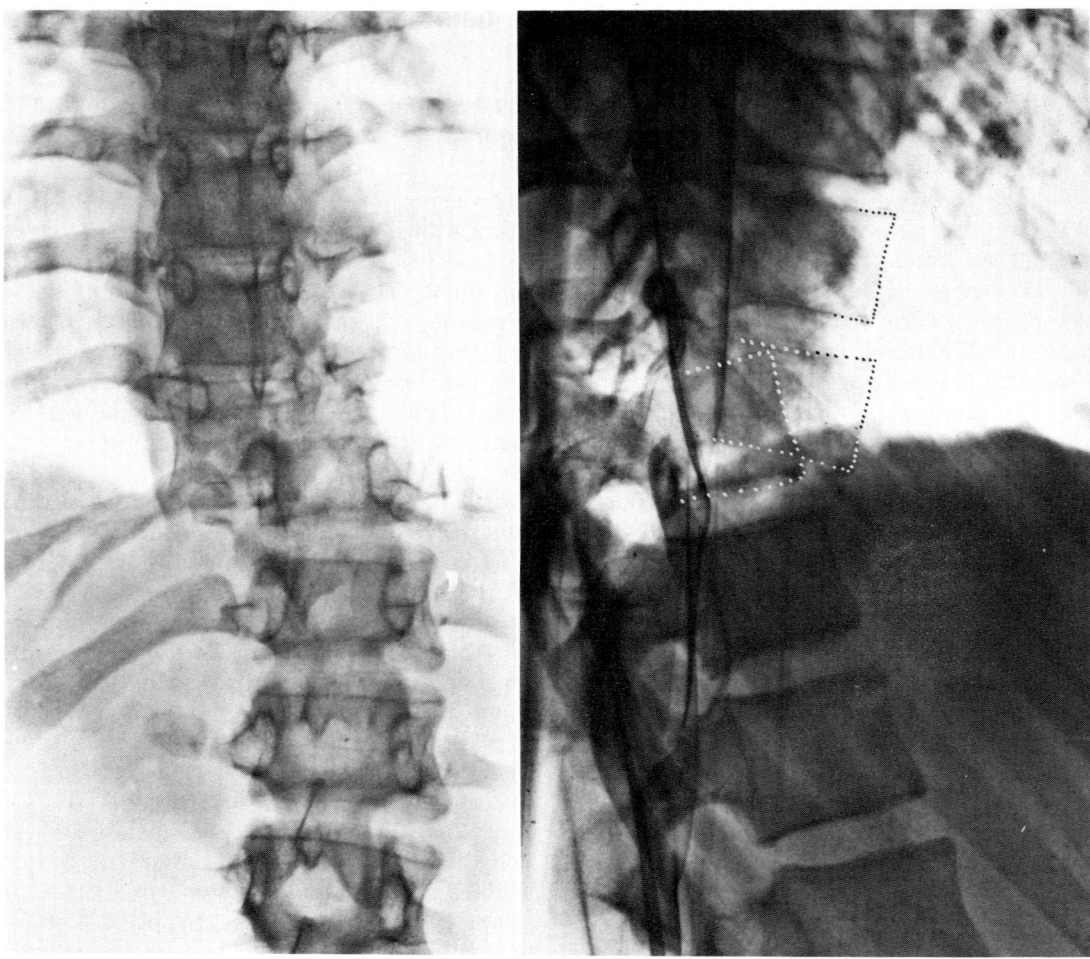

Fig. 1. Irreducible fracture dislocation of T 10/11 (patient B.M.; female; 16 years old).

MACNAB observed that a wedge fracture of the vertebra with more than 50% lowering of the anterior border of the vertebra automatically results in a major incongruity of the intervertebral joints, which leads to a spondyloarthrosis [112]. In the long term, a pronounced wedge fracture of the vertebra of the thoracolumbar junction can lead to Baastrup disease in addition to the compensatory hyperlordosis as shown in Figure 4. In addition, MORSCHER includes reduced spinal mobility, stress and age in the indications for surgery. The poorer the mobility of the spine and pre-existing kyphosis, for example in Scheuermann disease, the greater the occupational demands on the patients back, and the younger the adult patient, the more appropriate is internal fixation and fracture reduction [129, 130, 134, 137]. If pain unexpectedly occurs later on, the indications are similar, and a corrective osteotomy can eliminate the deformity in the healed fracture, but the patient then has to undergo the healing and rehabilitation phases twice (Fig. 5).

*d)* Surgery is indicated in patients with intracerebral trauma, athetosis, or in addiction, where adequate immobilization or fixation cannot be achieved by conservative measures, and secondary injury may occur due to uncontrolled ambulation (Fig. 6).

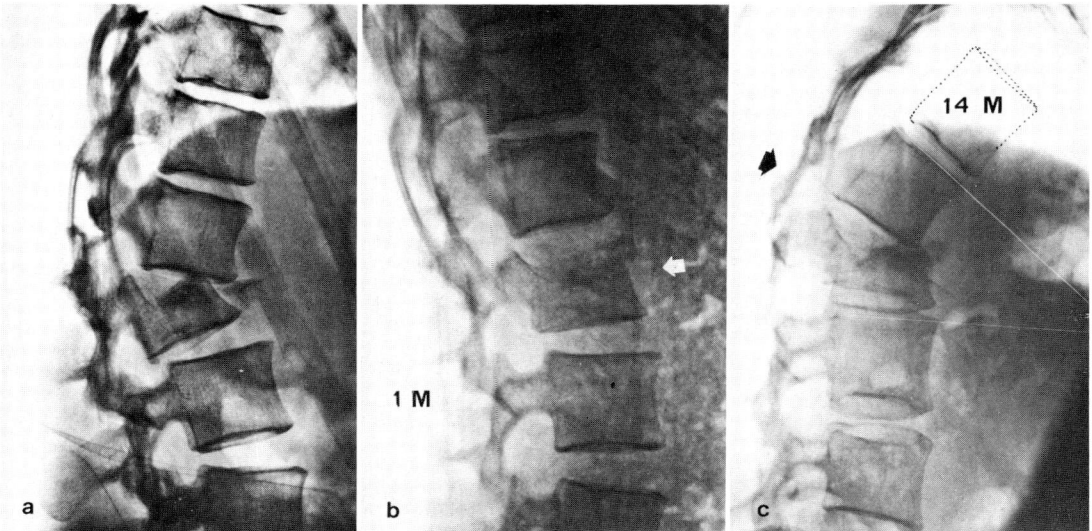

Fig. 2. Fracture dislocation of L1 with rupture of the posterior elements (patient B.A.; female 26 years old); a) radiograph on day of injury, b) after reduction during conservative treatment, c) 14 months post injury, persistent instability because of lack of tension band function of the torn posterior ligaments (see arrow).

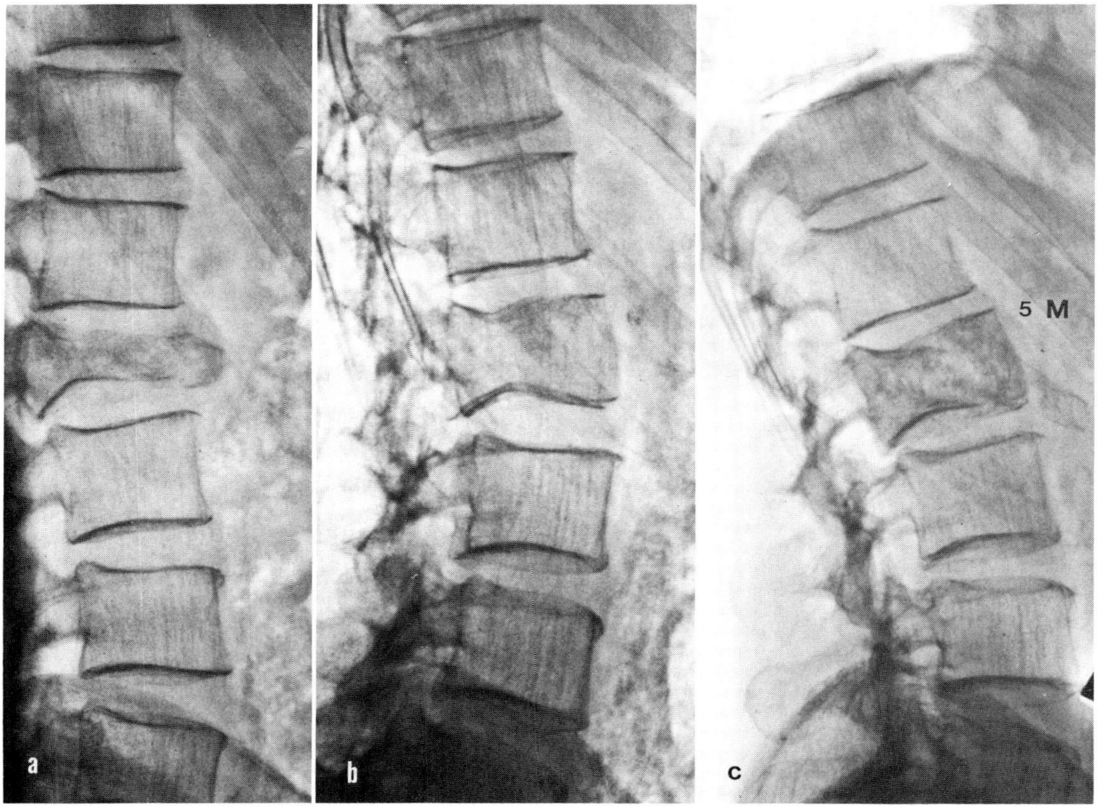

Fig. 3a. Fracture of L1 (patient H.E.; male; 55 years old); a) radiograph on day of injury, b) ten hours post reduction, c) five months post injury under conservative treatment with 12 weeks of bedrest; full mobilization without corset.

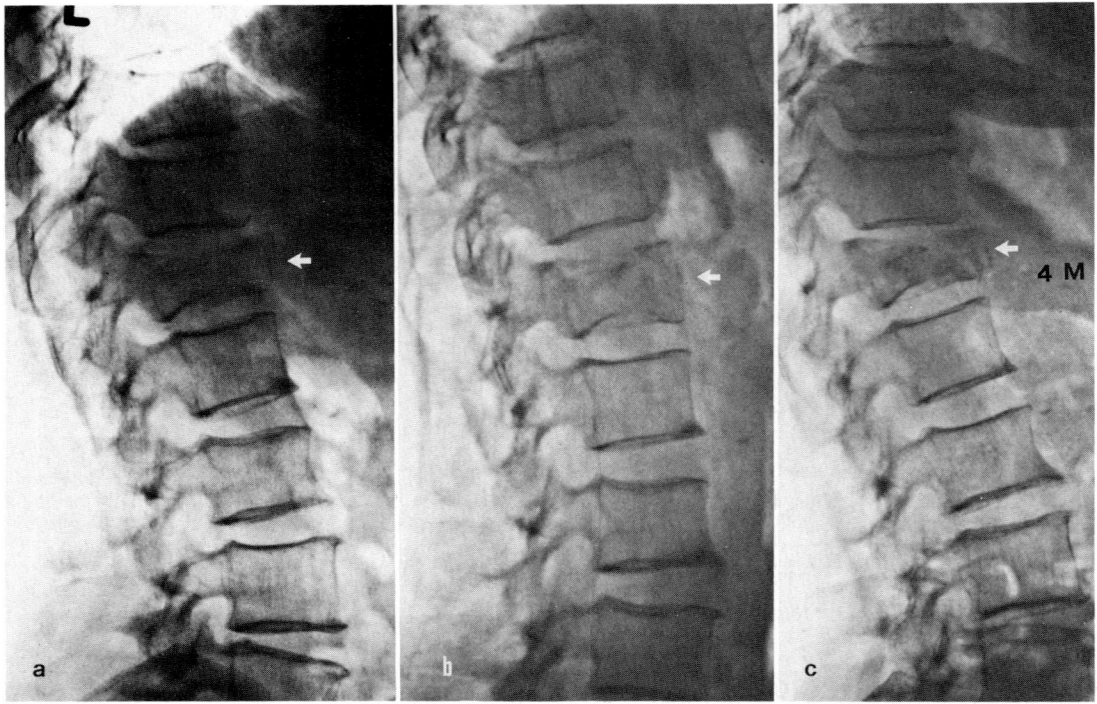

Fig. 3b. Fracture of T12 (patient K.M.; female; 69 years old); a) radiograph on the day of injury, b) five days after postural reduction, c) four months later under the same treatment as in the patient in Fig. 3a.

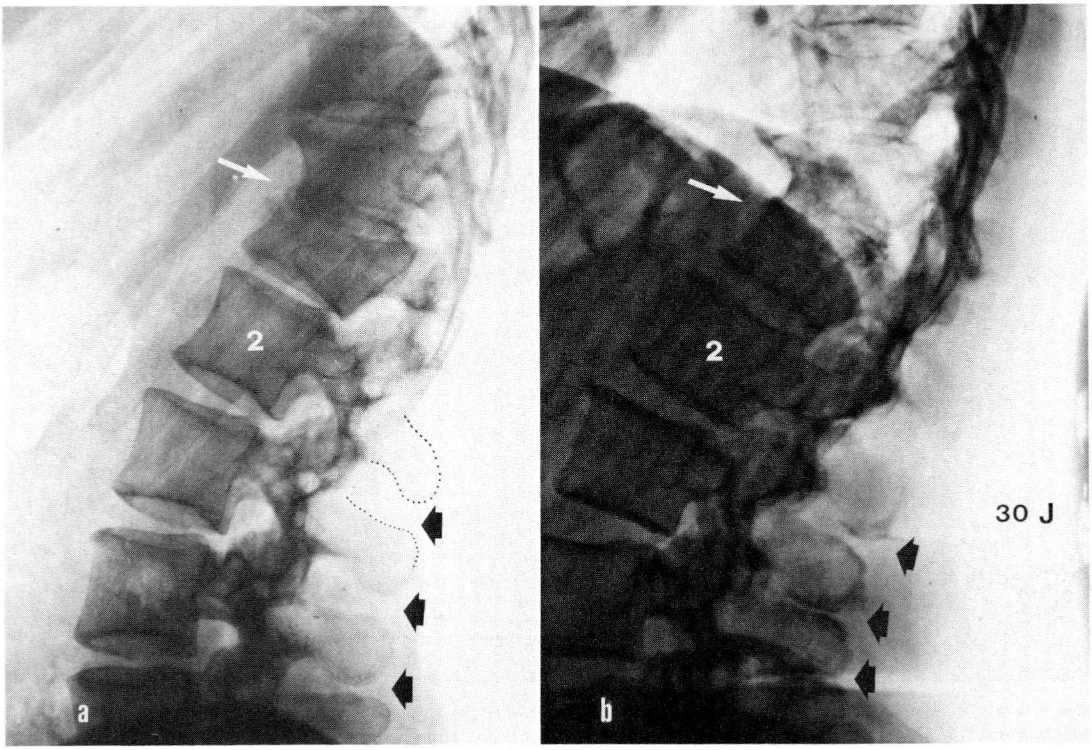

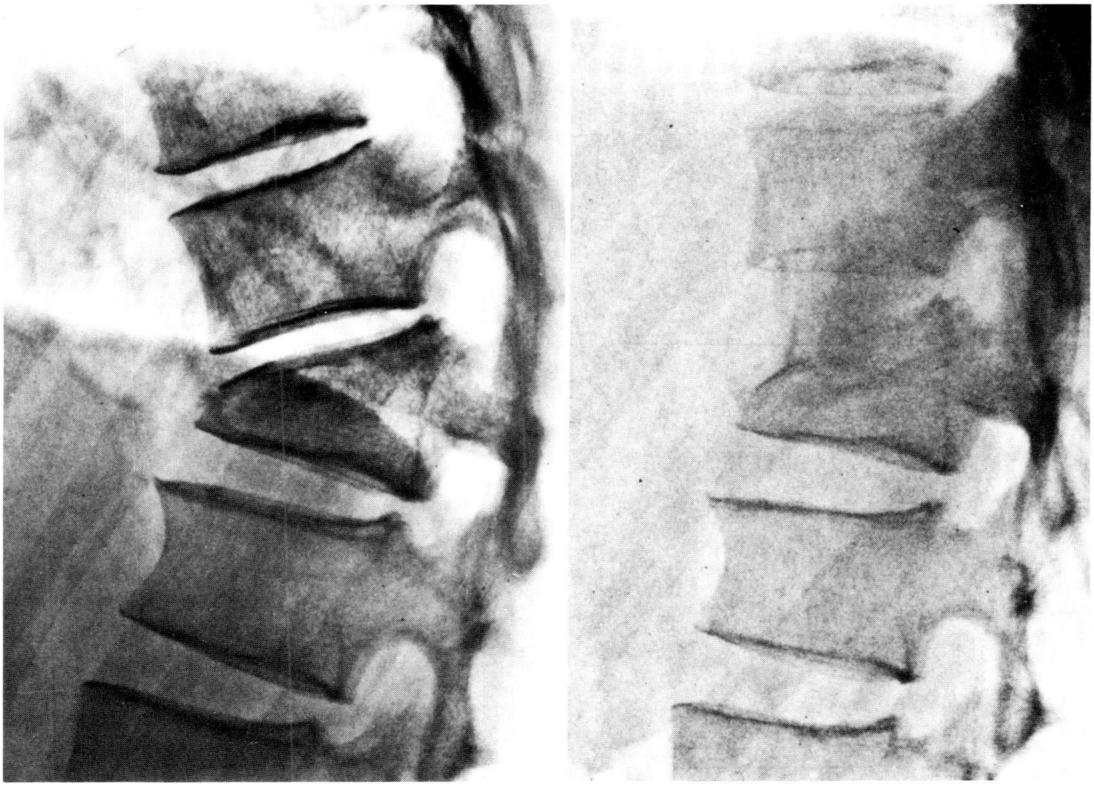

Fig. 5. Radiograph three years after fracture of L1 with 34 degrees of kyphosis and chronic pain at the compensatory lordosis and at the fracture site (patient D.M.; male; 40 years old); a) before corrective osteotomy of T12 and L1, b) one year after corrective osteotomy.

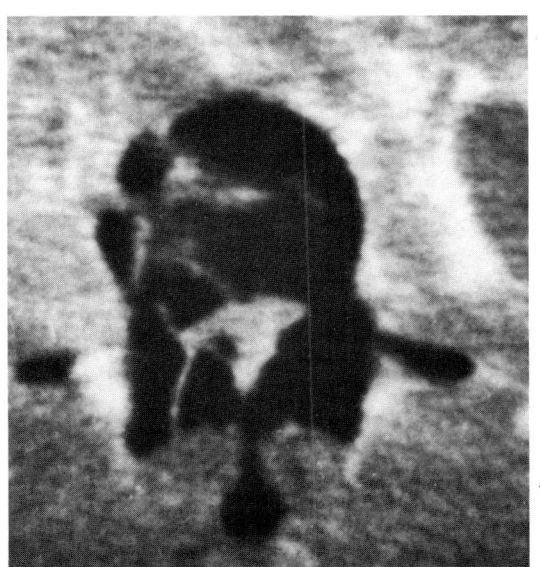

## 3.2 Vertebral fractures with neurological injury

The indications for surgical treatment discussed in section 1 apply equally to patients with transverse lesions of the spinal cord with paresis, because severe posttraumatic deformities can lead to long term structural symptoms and vertebral pain, and limit rehabilitation. Deformity or instability should be corrected despite the spinal cord lesion. However, there are additional indications for surgical intervention in neurological injuries:

◁ Fig. 6. Fracture of L2 in a patient with severe cerebral injury, little subluxation on plain films, but danger of secondary dislocation in a restless patient according to the CT findings (patient D.J.; 40 years old).

◁ Fig. 4. Fracture of L1 with 30 degrees of kyphosis (patient V.L.; female; 29 years old); a) radiograph on the day of injury, b) 30 years after injury, a Baastrup lesion has arisen owing to the compensatory hyperlordosis (see black arrows).

*e)* Where there is a time interval between the accident and the onset of the paralysis. These are cases of secondary paralysis where the trauma itself has not led to irreversible spinal or root lesions, but has arisen from secondary damage due, for example, to increased pressure or ischemia. In principle, the lesion in these cases may therefore be reversible if treated early. This is an indication for urgent surgery with reduction of the displacement and relief of pressure. For example, in cervical dislocation, immediate closed reduction can be performed, and there is then no urgency for subsequent stabilization.

*f)* Where there is progression of initially incomplete paralysis, the same applies as in e).

*g)* Open spinal cord injuries, which are most often caused by gunshot injuries, are always treated surgically [62]. Apart from gunshot injuries, these injuries are very rare. From 1000 cases at the Swiss Paraplegia Center in Basle, there was only one open injury. CLARK restricts surgery only to infected open injuries and treats other open injuries conservatively [27].

*h)* Incomplete transverse lesions in which there is no neurological recovery, or initial improvement stops at a plateau and in which there is a coincidental narrowing in the cross section of the vertebral canal. «Incomplete» means that the spinal cord is not destroyed irreversibly, and there is either only partial motor paralysis, or there is sparing of pain fibers in the sacral area, or the lesion has affected the peripheral nerves at the cauda equina rather than the spinal cord.

The currently accepted definition of irreversible spinal damage is that a complete transverse lesion of the spinal cord is present with loss of sacral sensation after the period of spinal shock, when there will be a return of the bulbocavernous reflex 24–48 hours after the injury. In the first 24–48 hours (when the bulbocavernosus reflex is still absent), it is impossible to assess spinal cord function properly. It has not yet been clarified with certainty from what degree a narrowing of the canal cross-section is significant; this also depends on the location level. At the thoracolumbar junction a 10 to 20% reduction of the spinal canal is probably significant.

GUTTMANN [63] and BEDBROOK [9] do not think that spinal canal narrowing is important, and point out that damage to the spinal cord is more dependent on the trauma with the resultant local biochemical and circulatory results. Although surgery has the advantage of restoring anatomy and shortening hospital treatment, as yet no statistical difference has been shown in the rate of neurological recovery between surgically and non-surgically treated patients [25, 33, 34, 43, 49, 78, 148, 217], even though it has been emphasised that patients with more severe spinal injury more commonly undergo surgical treatment [144]. Neurological damage secondary to surgery has also been reported (KEMPF et al. [93]: two cases out of 50, GERTZBEIN et al. [54]: one case out of 36, MALCOLM [122]: four cases out of 14). On the other hand, JACOBS et al.. [81], BOHLMANN and EISMONT [18], ROSENTHAL and LOWERY [162], MAGERL [115], ROY-CAMILLE et al. [165], LEWIS and McKIBBIN [103], VALENCAK et al. [197], BRADFORD et al. [25], FLESH et al. [49], OSEBOLD et al. [148], HOLDSWORTH [78], DICKSON et al. [43], YOSIPOVITCH et al. [217] did not find any increase of neurological symptoms after operation.

The word «operation» is defined in this work as reduction and stabilization of the spine alone or in addition to a laminectomy, since laminectomy without stabilization is unacceptable, because it does not allow a true decompression [30, 62, 63, 148]. Generally, the narrowing of the spinal canal occurs anteriorly due to anteriorly situated debris, intervertebral disc tissue, and the posterior edge of the subluxated vertebra; it also occurs as a result of the kyphosis. This leads to tension in the dorsal part of the dura, which thus presses the dural contents against the posterior wall of the vertebral body even if the arch has been removed dorsally. In addition, laminectomy sometimes increases the neurological damage, because it gives rise to additional instability and thus increases the kyphosis [149]. MORGAN et al. [128] found that 52% of patients with partial neurological injury deteriorated after surgery, and BOHLMANN [17] found this in five of 16 of his patients.

*i)* According to RUGE [169], other objectives of an operation are also the comfort of the patient and an early physical and occupational rehabilitation. Those situations in which surgical treatment provides a noteworthy increase in comfort (i. e. relief for the patient and no greater convenience for the nursing staff), or in which the operation entails an appreciable gain in time without deterioration in the final result are hence at least to be discussed as indications for surgery above and beyond the points a)–h). These are of course relative indications and depend to a large extent on the ability to achieve successfully the objectives of surgery without complications. Weighing up benefit against risk will always be a personal decision and will depend on the attitude and experience of the surgeon and the circumstances of the individual case, and cannot be standardized. However, there is little doubt that methods of surgical treatment for fractures of the thoracolumbar spine must be improved first, unlike the situation in the cervical spine where the advantages of surgical stabilization are widely accepted (see section 1.1).

The interest of the patient in early physical rehabilitation gains significance in an other way: this is the costs of our hospital system, which make it imperative to reduce the duration of the patient's stay in hospital. This should not be at the cost of the rehabilitation phase, but may only involve the initial period of bedrest [37].

### 3.3 Impending vertebral fractures (tumor surgery)

Within the skeletal system, the spine is most commonly affected by tumor metastases [87]. BARRON et al. showed that in tumor cases the most frequent cause of spinal cord compression, apart from extradural tumor masses and intradural metastases, was pressure from pathological fracture dislocations and from angular kyphoses. Radiotherapy or chemotherapy alone are not adequate to treat these complications [22]. Spinal cord injury can be prevented by mechanical stabilization [168] or by surgical reduction, decompression by tumor resection and stabilization of the spine, where the pathological fracture has just occurred but as yet not resulted in a complete paraplegia. Naturally the same applies to the rare primary spinal tumors which have led to mechanical weakening.

The indications for surgical treatment of vertebral fractures can thus be extended beyond those in sections 3.1 and 3.2:

*k)* prophylaxis in vertebral metastases or primary tumors of the spine in which pathological fracture is impending, either directly due to the osteolytic process or due to the tumor resection or surgical decompression.

Preconditions for surgery are that the tumor is operable and that surgery is suitable in terms of the patient's life expectancy and quality of life. The appraisal of this depends to a great extent on the basic attitude of the treating physican to advanced tumors, and it is always possible to criticise management decisions in any individual case retrospectively. However, if it is possible to preserve walking ability to the end and to prolong survival time by several months [168, 176], surgery is justified. Stabilization should always be accompanied by resection of as much as possible of the accessible tumor mass. Surgical technique will differ from case to case and depends on the main site of tumor involvement; anterior and posterior techniques are to be considered in these cases [22, 65, 67, 176].

It is difficult to be sure in any one case whether a pathological fracture is imminent; NATHER and BOSE [142] did not have any cases of instability in the follow up examination of their 39 patients with spinal metastases who had been decompressed dorsally by laminectomy without additional stabilization in any case. Two out of 23 of our patients who underwent operation for pathological fracture presented with the fracture as the first symptom of metastasis.

## 4. Stabilization techniques

### 4.1 Pure osteosyntheses

Pure osteosyntheses (i.e. fixation of fragments of a single bone with restoration of anatomy) are only applicable in a few types of spinal fracture, for example simple detachment fractures of the transverse processes or spinous processes, where there is no real indication for surgery anyway. Thus there remain only two types of fracture in which pure osteosynthesis has any place. These are both in the cervical spine, namely internal screw fixation of a fresh dens fracture [11, 12] and screw osteosynthesis of the arch in the «hangman fracture» [118, 197, 204]. In the thoracolumbar spine, the only real indication for osteosynthesis is in pars interarticularis spondylolysis of the lumbar spine, if spondylolysis due to microtrauma is to be counted as a type of fracture.

### 4.1.1 Screw fixation of the pars interarticularis of the vertebral arch in the lumbar spine

Stabilization of the pars interarticularis with a hook screw as described by MORSCHER [136] is a type of compression osteosynthesis. The arch of the affected vertebra is exposed subperiosteally starting from the spinous process. The area of spondylolysis can easily be identified due to the instability of the dorsal arch which is visible once it has been freed of connective tissue. The proximal part of the pedicle with the cranial articular facet becomes visible in the depth. It is covered dorsally by the distal articular facet of the more proximal vertebra. If this articular process is especially long as is often the case, it is shortened. Since it is possible that the spondylolysis is caused by its chisel action on the pars interarticularis in hyperextension. A special screw[1] is introduced into the cranial articular process of the affected vertebra immediately caudal to the intervertebral joint. It is anchored in bone with its 20 mm long cancellous bone thread leaving the unthreaded part of the screw outside the bone. A hook from the instrument set is then mounted on the shaft of the screw, hooked around the lytic arch, and put under compression by means of a nut on the counterthread of the screw shaft. The screw does not pass through the zone of spondylolysis, but beside it and allows excellent visualization during introduction of the screw, and also enables the defect to be filled with cancellous bone. Postoperatively, an orthopedic lumbar corset is used for six to 12 months. The progressive ossification of the spondylolysis is apparent in oblique radiographs (Fig. 7). This procedure is only indicated in adolescents under 18 years old. In older patients, intervertebral disc degeneration is usually already present and this can give rise to pain, even after stabilization of the spondylolysis.

### 4.2 Stabilization and spondylodesis

In all other fractures, restoration of the shape of the individual broken vertebra ad integrum with simultaneous load-bearing capacity is not possible with surgical stabilization. The aim of surgery is to achieve a satisfactory spinal con-

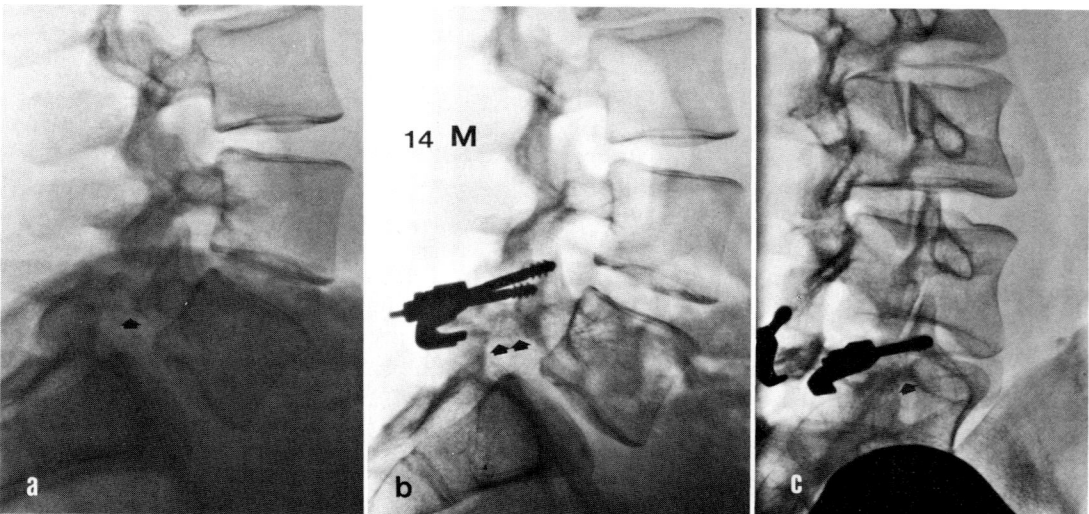

Fig. 7. L5 spondylolysis (patient W.C.; female; 18 years old); a) a clear area of lysis of the pars interarticularis is visible preoperatively in the lateral radiograph (see arrow), b) 14 months postoperatively; screws have been introduced cranially outside the pars interarticularis into the proximal articular process of L5, the hooks holding the arch of L5. The area of lysis has consolidated (see arrows), c) oblique radiograph 14 months postoperatively.

[1] Firm R. Mathys, Surgical Instrument Manufacturer, CH–2544 Bettlach, Switzerland.

figuration that will allow axial loading. Movement between the injured vertebra and at least one adjacent vertebra will be lost in order to achieve spinal stability with surgery. In most stabilization procedures, a number of further vertebrae with healthy intervertebral joints need to be included at least temporarily in the arthrodesis, in order to obtain satisfactory achoring of implants and to allow the biomechanics of the fixation to act. Hence any gain from surgery in each case should be balanced against the inevitable loss of function.

### 4.2.1 Dorsal procedures

#### 4.2.1.1 *Distracting procedures*

*Harrington distraction instrumentation:* Harrington distraction instrumentation which is widely used in scoliosis surgery has achieved widespread application in the surgical treatment of thoracic and lumbar fractures, with rods being placed bilaterally. When used in fracture reduction and stabilization, the biomechanical action of the implant is changed, and thus the loading has been altered. An understanding of this alteration is important in order to decide on the indications for application, and also to explain the difficulties which sometimes occur. In fracture treatment, where the vertebral arch is preserved, there is effectively a three-point bending moment, whereas there is a four-point bending moment when the vertebral arch is destroyed. The cranial and caudal hooks exert a posterior force on the corresponding vertebral arches two to three segments away from the fractured vertebra, whereas the intermediate part of the rod exerts an anterior force on the fractured vertebra where the arch is preserved, or on the adjacent arches where the vertebral arch is fractured (see Fig.9). Thus the system corrects kyphosis of the fractured spine. However, so

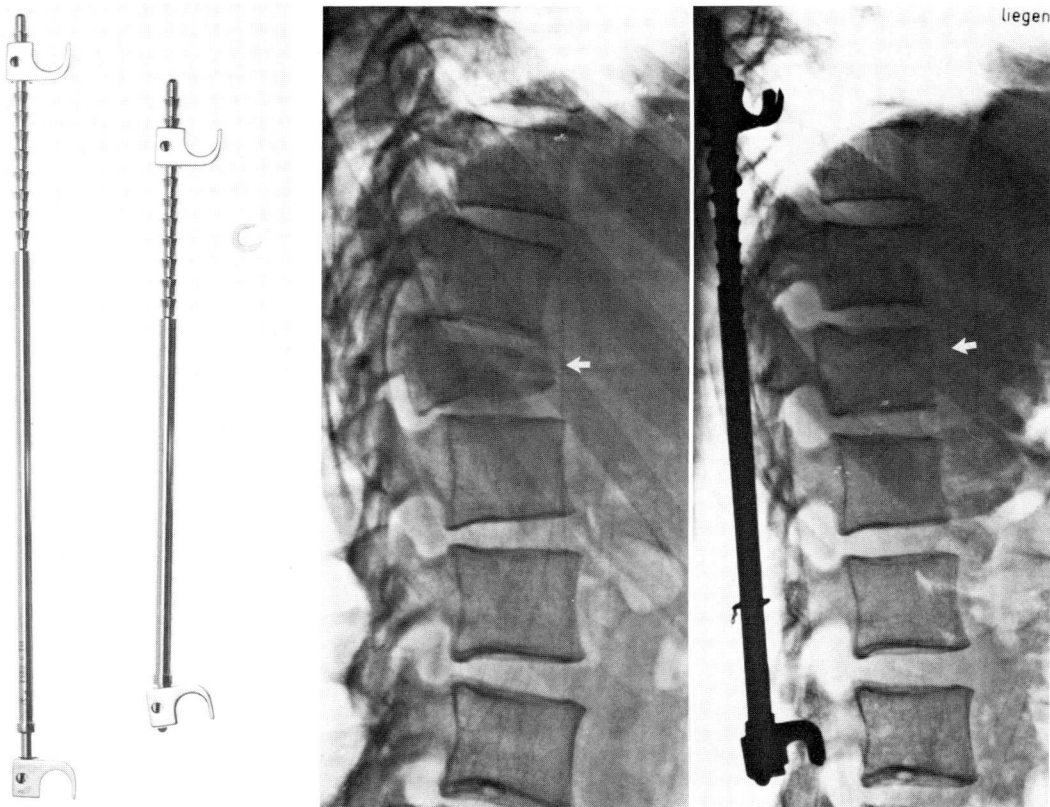

Fig. 8. Fracture of L 1 reduced with Harrington distraction instrumentation four hours post injury. The preserved ligamentous complex has repositioned the posterior wall of the fractured vertebra.

21

that the laminae remain within the hooks and do not slide out, distraction of the system is necessary. In order to make distraction effective for securing the hook position in spite of the posteriorly acting force, there must be a firm ligamentous resistance against which the system can be distracted [4].

The distraction force has an immediate effect on the fractured vertebra, and can restore its height. In addition, repositioning of the fracture fragments may occur in both the AP and lateral view in burst fractures where the longitudinal ligaments are intact, because traction leads to increased periosteal tension as in a tube, as shown in Figure 8.

WHITE, PANJABI and THOMAS [209] characterized the intensity and direction of forces which occur on the kyphotic spine when using distraction instrumentation, as shown in Figure 9.

In order for Harrington distraction instrumentation to be effective, the intact vertebral arches must have direct contact with the distraction rods, so that these can transmit the anterior reducing force. However, this does not occur initially in the lumbar spine, until the distraction force leads to elimination of the lordosis, at which point the vertebral arches make contact with the rods. Only then does four-point fixation occur.

The point of action of the distraction force on the laminae is situated posterior to the instantaneous axis of rotation of the vertebra; thus distraction results in slight kyphosis of the terminal vertebra.

There is no doubt that excellent clinical results can be obtained with the Harrington distraction instrumentation as long as it is properly applied, the indications are correct, and adequate follow-up occurs, as shown in the extensive literature

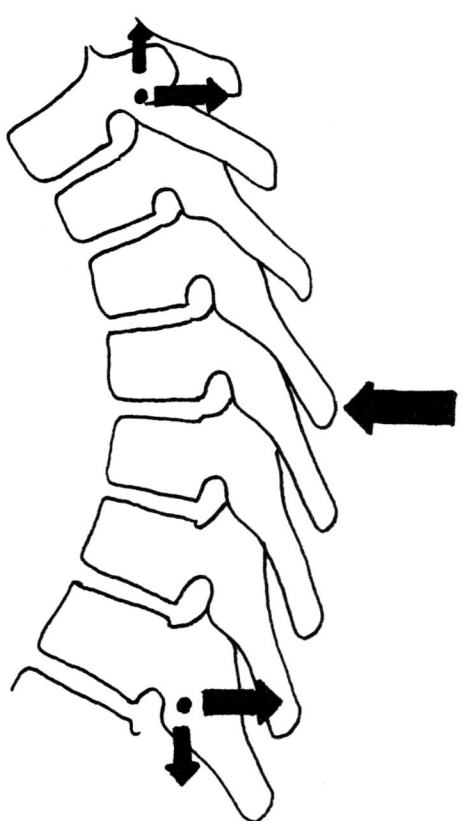

Fig. 9. The forces occurring with Harrington distraction instrumentation as described by WHITE et al. [209].

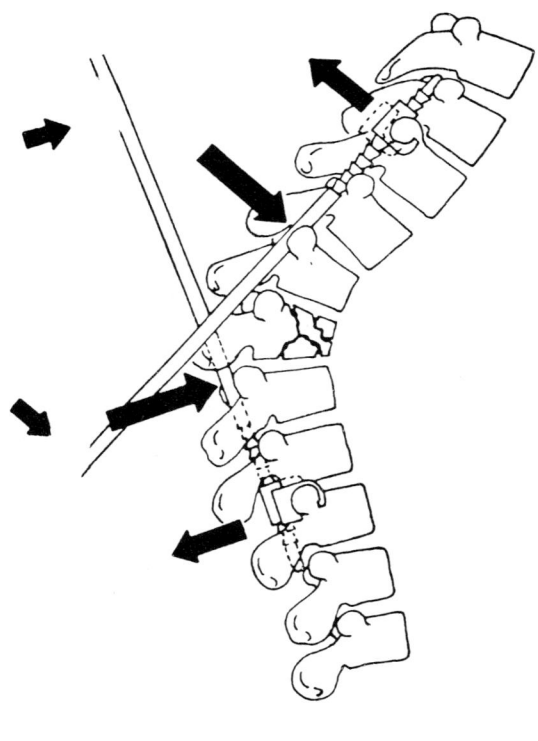

Fig. 10. Reduction maneuver as described by WHITE et al. [209] with inverted distraction rods in kyphosis.

[25, 29, 43, 46, 49, 54, 71, 93, 148, 162, 200, 210, 217]. The simple surgical technique is without doubt a major advantage. The seating for the distal hooks is created by removal of the ligamentum flavum with a minimum of bone resection. If the space between the vertebral arches is too small, bone can be resected from the proximal arch in order not to weaken the arch carrying the hook, otherwise fracturing may occur in loading [54]. Placing the proximal hook in the thoracic region, it is often helpful to cut the lower edge of the lamina transversely and medially after excision of the ligamentum flavum, in order to counteract the tendency of the hook to migrate laterally. For the same reason, the hook should be placed under the lamina and not between the joint facets [54] and not against the pedicle. Use of the outrigger is usually not appropriate since three-point fixation cannot be exerted. Using simultaneously bilateral Harrington rods a forceful three-point bending moment occurs. WHITE et al. [209] suggest that one rod can be inverted upside down as shown in Figure 10. In the

thoracic region, prebending of the rods may be necessary in a severe pre-existing kyphosis.

The problems which occur with Harrington distraction instrumentation can be explained once its biomechanical action is understood.

1. The system requires resistance to be tightened, and the best anatomical structures to resist distraction are the two posterior columns [83]. If there is ligamentous continuity, the laminae are held securely in the hooks by distraction, and this is the best indication for Harrington distraction instrumentation. However, when the system is used in complete discontinuity of the posterior columns, the only structure under tension will be the anterior longitudinal ligament, and the distance between the posterior elements may increase with forward inclination of the trunk, so that the rods can detach from the hooks (Fig. 11) or the hooks can detach from the laminae. For those cases, compression instrumentation would be biomechanically better but is often not feasible because there is simultaneous fracture of the posterior wall of the vertebral body.

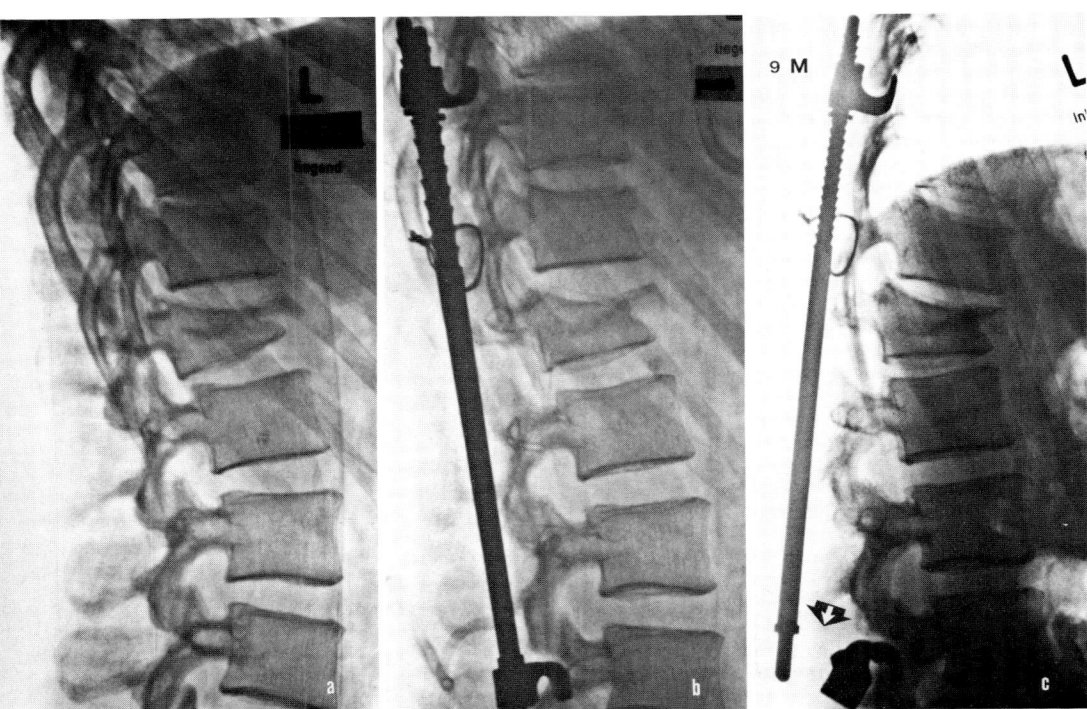

Fig. 11. Fracture of L1, treated with Harrington distraction rods with the «three vertebrae above, three vertebrae below» technique (patient L.M.; male; 26 years old); a) lordosis position, b) postoperative radiograph shows only incomplete reduction c) nine months post injury, rods detached distally from the hooks during flexion of the spine.

Therefore in postoperative treatment additional external support is indicated preventing forward flexion, for example a plaster jacket, a polypropylene double corset etc. This should be worn for up to 20 weeks [43, 49, 54, 217].

2. On the basis of three-point bending moments, the cranial hook exerts a posterior force on the lamina. The inner surface of the lamina runs obliquely anteriorly from its lower edge. If the vertebra tilts anteriorly, this surface will become increasingly more horizontal, and the part of the lamina held by the hook will become smaller until ultimately it is no longer stable. The hook will then either cut out fracturing the lamina, or slip out without fracture [153].

Hook detachments are reported clinically as one of the commonest complications [29, 43, 54], and in laboratory tests the «mode of failure» is almost always hook detachment with or without damage to the edge of the lamina as shown in Figure 12 [153, 186, 214].

Anterior tilting of the instrumented vertebra may arise when the fractured body collapses, if the upper hook is placed too near to the fracture. In WÖRSDÖRFER's experiments [214] the hooks detached under forward flexion loading when a kyphosis of 3.50 was reached at the fractured segment itself, tilting of the instrumented vertebra two segments higher being much greater. Anterior tilting may also arise due to the small gap between the indentations of the distraction rod and the next vertebral arch. According to JACOBS et al. [81], a 4 mm gap will cause tilting of 10° until the arch meets the rod, when instrumentation is performed in the «two vertebrae above, two vertebrae below the fracture» manner as recommended by FLESH et al. [49].

JACOBS et al. [81] recommend the use of a long rod as a remedy, following the rule of «three vertebrae above, three vertebrae below». This appreciably reduces the possibility of tilting, and also doubles the lever arm of «hook/next arch»

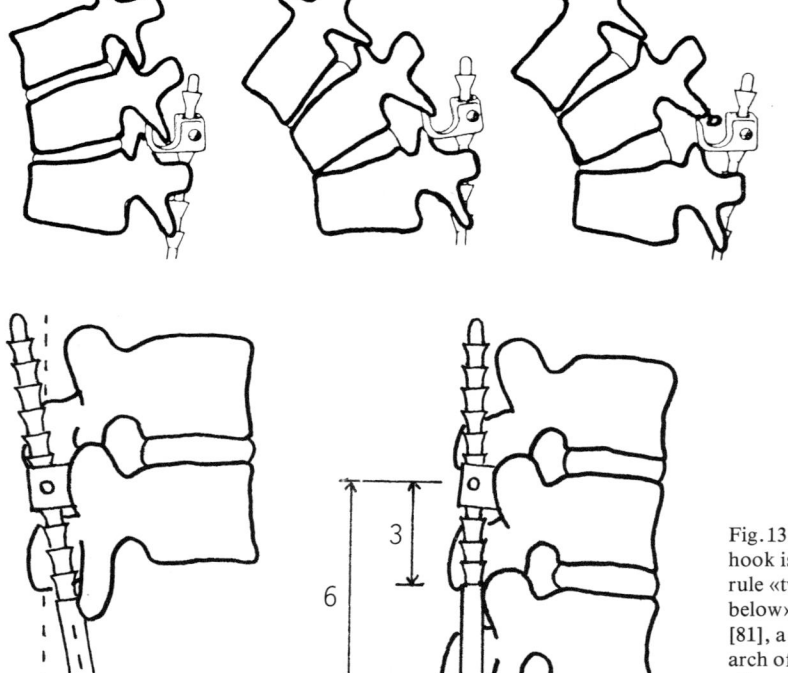

Fig. 12. Detachment of cranial Harrington hook, associated with tilting of the vertebra rendering the lamina more horizontal (PURCELL et al. [153]).

Fig. 13. Where the upper Harrington hook is placed in accordance with the rule «two vertebrae above, two vertebrae below», as described by JACOBS et al. [81], a 4 mm gap between the rod and the arch of the vertebra below is sufficient to allow tilting of the vertebra by 10°. The tilt is very much less using the technique of «three vertebrae above, three vertebrae below». In addition, the forces are halved by doubling the lever arm.

from about 3 cm, to «hook/next arch but one» to 6 cm. The forces acting on the bone are thus reduced by half (Fig.13). In an experimental study, JACOBS et al. [83] were able to show that when applying the fixation three vertebrae above and three vertebrae below the injury, it had double the energy absorption and approximately three times the load carrying capacity before the hooks cut out, when compared with fixation using two vertebrae above and two vertebrae below the injury.

PURCELL et al. [153] showed that by placing the upper hooks three vertebrae above the unstable segment and two vertebrae below, they were able to double the load carrying capacity experimentally. Hence they suggested the application of the hooks «three vertebrae above, two vertebrae below» in clinical practice.

3. As mentioned above, the three point fixation of the rods requires contact between the rods and the vertebral arches. For the rod to be effective, it must be shaped to fit the final contour of the spine. In the lumbar region, the rod would need to be contoured into lordosis. However, this is not possible with the normal Harrington rod, because the rod can rotate 180° in the hooks as soon as a kyphotic force occurs, resulting in severe kyphosis. In order to solve this problem,

rods with a square lower end and corresponding hooks with a square hole were developed, and this allows the rods to be bent in a lordotic configuration.

4. The three-point fixation of the rod leads to an appreciable bending force on the distraction rod which was originally designed mainly for axial forces. DICKSON et al. [43] reported rod breakages in 6% of cases. The greatest angulation on the rod occurs in the middle of the rod, and the greatest tension at the first notch. In the notch the diameter of the rod is 4.75 mm, the full cross section being 6.35 mm. NEUGEBAUER [143] calculated experimentally that a rod of the same diameter without the notches would withstand forces three times as great. At the site of force transmission from the hook into the rod, the strain is very much less than in the middle of the rod.

An attempt has been made to solve this problem by using a longer length Harrington rod such that the hook comes to rest in the lowest notch, and the more cranial part of the rod is resected [143]. This leads to difficulties in surgical technique because the spreading pliers cannot be used initially in placing the rod; however, these problems are soluble. By applying the rods in this way, the site of the greatest

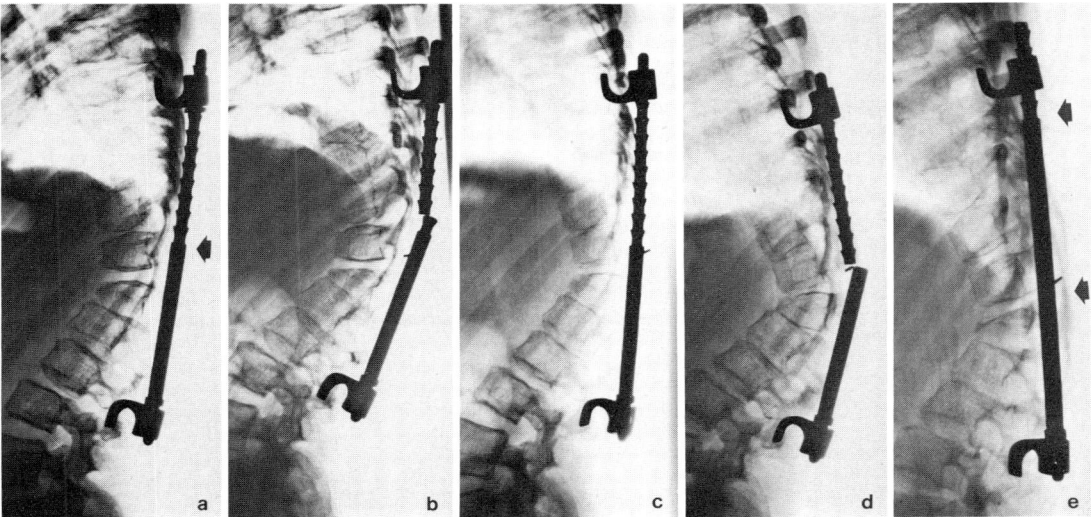

Fig. 14. Kyphoscoliosis after laminectomy in early childhood because of intradural tumor (patient S. J., female, 11 years old). Weakest point of the rod and the greatest bending strain coincide (arrow). Break of the rod occurs twice after an interval of 18 months (b–d). By choosing a long rod which is shortened above the hook, the main bending strain and the weakest point of the rod are separated (arrows, Fig. e). At the end of growth an anterior corrective fusion was performed.

bending strain «at the middle of the rod», and the lowest load carrying capacity (the first notch) are as far apart as possible (Fig. 14). Naturally, the part of the rod projecting above the hook must be shortened.

5. Two technical problems using Harrington instrumentation for spinal trauma should be mentioned. Firstly, the distance of the notches (6.4 mm) is large, and not uncommonly the desired distraction would be between the two notches. Secondly, the loose connection between the hook and the rod does not allow any rotational fixation. The experimental work of WÖRSDÖRFER [216] shows that the fracture fragments are distracted with the Harrington instrumentation, so that osseous interdigitation of the fracture surfaces is distracted, and this further decreases the rotational stability present before instrumentation. This is of course not a problem in scoliosis surgery, but for use in trauma cases, rotational stability would be important. These two problems cannot be countered by tricks in surgical technique.

*Locking hook spinal rod system* (Fig. 15): In 1979, JACOBS et al. [84] presented a further development of the Harrington distraction instrumentation set which is claimed to produce a better solution for the problems mentioned in sections 2–5 above. The following changes were made:

– Instead of notches, both ends of the rods are provided with threads, so that linear distraction of any distance is possible, and weakening of the rod due to the narrow cross section occurring at the notches is avoided.

– The hooks fixed with the locking nuts are freely rotatable on the rod, but have a radial serration at one end, which engages with an identical serration on a washer. The shape of the washer does not allow rotation of the washer at the threaded part of the rod which is flattened on both sides, and thanks to the interdigitating teeth the hooks can be secured with rotational stability in steps of six degrees by tightening the nuts. The nuts also have a collar which can be crimped against the flattened sides of the rod once the nuts have been tightened, thus preventing loosening of the nuts. In this way, the rod can be contoured to the shape of the spine even in lordosis since rotation cannot occur, and hence the rod can lie against the vertebral arch. There is also rotational stability of the proximal and distal hooks.

– The diameter of the rod is raised to 7 mm, taking into account the large bending strain in the system when three-point fixation is used for fracture reduction.

– The lip of the cranial hook is tilted 15° away from the axis of the rod, and is thus shaped precisely to the anatomical shape of the anterior part of the proximal vertebral arch. In addition, the upper hook is fitted with a cover which can be pushed forward and which is secured by corresponding grooves on the upper part of the hook, and this can grip around the upper edge of the lamina or can be hammered into the lamina itself, if the lamina is too wide. When the hook nuts are tightened, the cover is also fixed, thus increasing the firm hold of the cranial hook (Fig. 16).

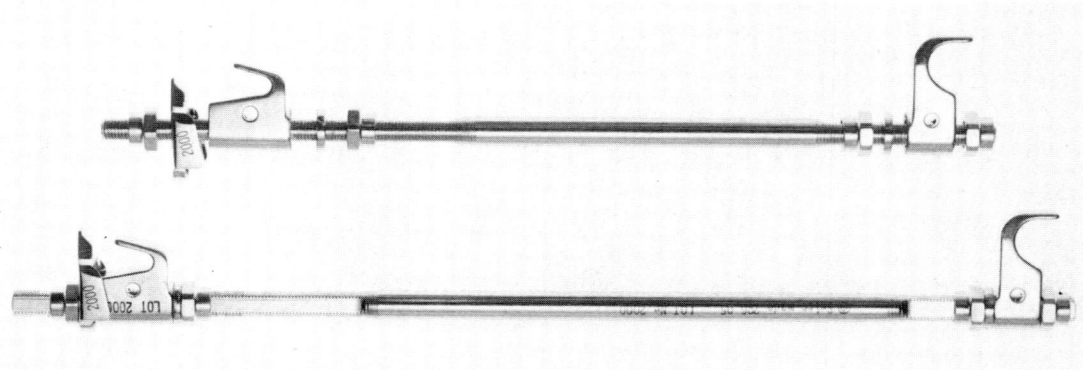

Fig. 15. Locking hook spinal rod system described by JACOBS [84].

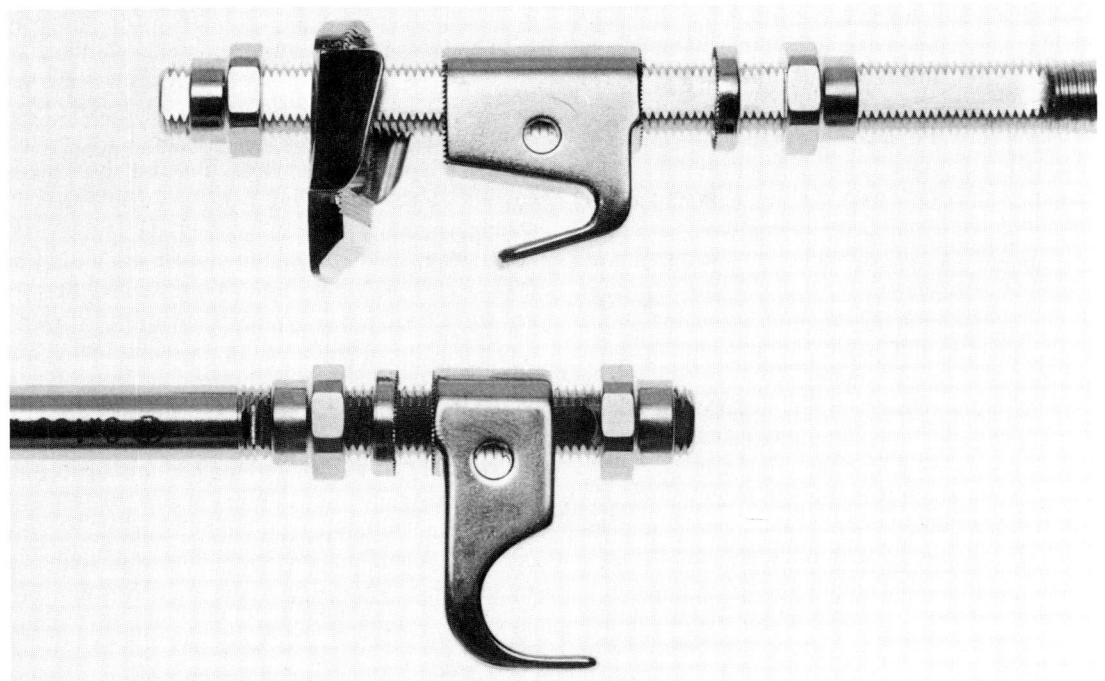

Fig. 16. Details of hook fixation.

First the placement of the hooks is prepared. After contouring the rod, the complete mounted system is implanted by inserting the caudal hook first. Then the fracture is reduced, and the cranial hook is driven upwards, sliding its lip under the lamina. The desired distraction using the nuts is then applied. The cover of the upper hook is put in position and the nuts are all tightened. Crimping together the collar of the nuts against the flattened rod prevents the nuts loosening. However the metal is soft enough to enable the nuts to be loosened using the wrench. JACOBS et al. [84] recommend implantation in accordance with the «three vertebrae above, three vertebrae below» rule, and have shown a 50% increase in the detachment force for the upper hook, and a threefold increase in stiffness in flexion of the instrumented lumbar spine using this kind of fixation [82]. WÖRSDÖRFER [214] measured the fixation using «two vertebrae above, two vertebrae below», which he regards as sufficient for this system. He found that a bending moment averaging 19.3 Nm was required before detachment of the upper hooks occurred. Interestingly then the same kyphotic deformation of about 3.6° occurred in the injured segment as in the experiments using the Harrington distraction system. However, roughly three times the bending moment was applied to obtain this deformity (the angular tilting of the terminal vertebra on the hook was of course greater than 3.6°). The objective of the major increase in stability is thus attained using the locking hook distraction instrumentation, although hook detachments may still occur. However, the main disadvantage of both systems is the length of the fixation distance and this is discussed separately in chapter 5.

*External fixator:* The external fixator [113] introduced by MAGERL in 1977 for the treatment of vertebral fractures allows distraction and stabilization without requiring three-point fixation (or four-point fixation), because the connection to the bone is not mobile via hooks, but is immobile via long Schanz' screws firmly fixed in the bone. These are screwed into the vertebral bodies through the pedicles, and their ends project percutaneously. Despite the long lever arms, it is possible to link them together with sufficient stability using the external fixator. The system can fix the position of the instrumented vertebrae in any desired position. By anchoring the screws in the vertebrae, leverage is not necessary on intact arches of adjacent vertebrae. Thus only the two vertebrae immediately adjacent to the fractured vertebra are instrumented. The spinal fixation extends only over two motion segments [117, 119] instead of over 4,5 or 6 segments as in the Harrington or locking-hook distraction instrumentation, depending on the implantation technique.

Since the direction of the Schanz' screws is given by the anatomical conditions of the narrow pedicle and is not adaptable, the external fixator must allow free adjustability in all directions. The frame developed by MAGERL and SCHLÄPFER fulfills this requirement with a high intrinsic stability [214], and enables a parallel distraction or compression force as well as lordotic or kyphotic tilting of the instrumented vertebrae via three threaded rods situated in ball and socket joints (Fig. 17). Thus exact reduction of the frac-

ture and subsequent mobilization of the patient with the external fixator frame is possible. Experience has shown that the fixation must be continued for four or five months until there is adequate consolidation of the fracture. The entire system displays high elasticity, and thus peak strains at the anchorage sites of the Schanz' screws in the bone are avoided. WÖRSDÖRFER [214] never saw detachment of the screws in experimental stability tests. He showed elastic deformation of the system with a return to the initial position using bending moments of up to 60 Nm, and a plastic deformation of the screws at even higher bending moments. MAGERL did not observe any screw extrusion in clinical use in his 49 cases [119]. Elasticity leads to movement at the fracture site, but clinical experience shows that these movements do not impair fracture healing. When the system is mounted without prestressing, alteration in the angle of kyphosis was found to be 2.5° at the fracture site, compared with 1.4° using osteosynthesis with dorsal plates, and 1.5° using the locking-hook distraction instruments in experiments where a bending

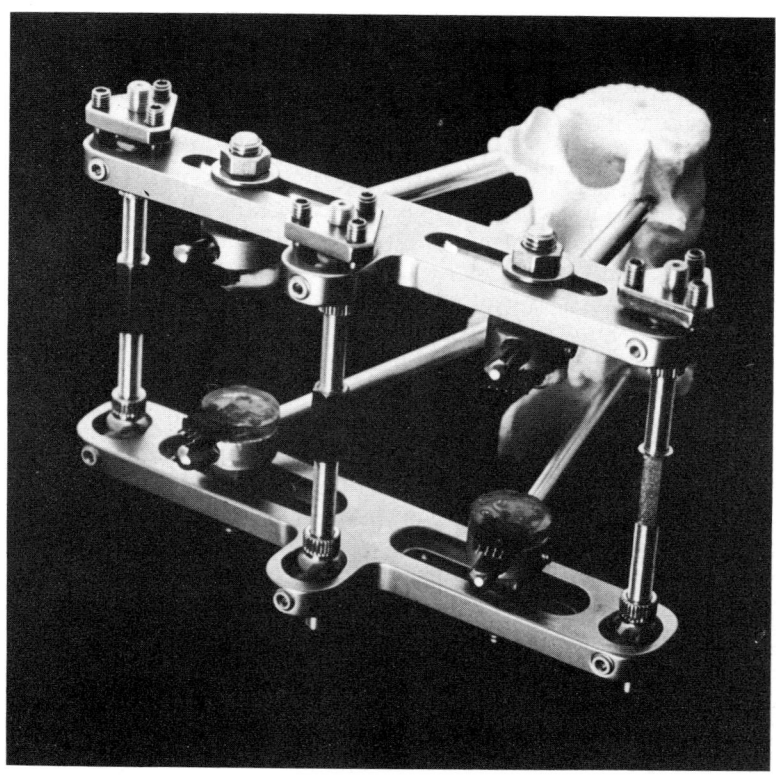

Fig. 17. External fixator described by MAGERL [116] and SCHLÄPFER [173].

moment of 10 Nm was applied. The Harrington distraction instrumentation tears out with loads less than this. All these experiments have been carried out in spinal specimens with combined anterior and posterior instability [214].

The advantages of the external fixator are obvious: very marked shortening of the fixation distance, high anchorage stability in the bone, no bulky implants and thus much space for substantial bone grafts, applicability in low lumbar fractures and very simple percutaneous removal without a second operation or anesthesia.

The disadvantages are less of a medical nature (according to MAGERL [117, 119], superficial infection, pin trac inflammation with spontaneous healing), but tend rather to concern psychological aspects («rods projecting from the back for five months»…) and above all the practicability: for paraplegics, both nursing and sitting in a normal wheelchair are made more difficult. Patients require especially adapted mattresses with a hole for the fixator and must wear a protective corset for the fixator. Thus the external fixator has only been used to a limited extent despite its tempting biomechanical principles.

### 4.2.1.2 Tension banding techniques

The center of gravity of the body is in front of the spine, which results in a flexion force. The mechanism of action of the vertebral column can hence be compared with that of a crane. Anteriorly there is a pressure-stressed column, consisting of the vertebral bodies and the intervertebral discs. Posteriorly there is a suspension system under tensile strain, consisting of the intersegmental ligaments of the vertebral arches and processes, the two columns of dorsal vertebral joints with their capsules and the erector musculature. Following the general principle that an injury is treated at the site of the defect to restore functional loss, it is logical to eliminate a traumatic disruption of the dorsal tensile system of the spine by an tension banding implant posteriorly, whereas the compression forces are resisted by the anterior bony column.

Disruptions of the dorsal tensile system occur either in isolation or in combination with anterior injuries. Isolated posterior injuries include fractures such as the «CHANCE fracture» [61], articular process fractures or pure ligamentous injuries in luxations. These injuries may also occur in combination with a wide range of anterior lesions from small anterior wedge compression fractures of the vertebral bodies to comminuted vertebral body fractures or complete ruptures of all the anterior structures. That injuries of the vertebral column with *intact* dorsal structures are very frequent is only to be mentioned here as a marginal note, as this type of injury is treated mainly using distraction methods.

HOLDSWORTH [76, 77, 78], ROAF [158] and JACOBS et al. [81] have analysed injury mechanism and fracture types. In practice, combinations of axial distraction, axial compression, flexion and rotation are frequently encountered.

As mentioned above, the anterior column must be able to resist compression forces when a posterior compression system is used, and this must be confirmed beforehand. It is generally agreed that the posterior wall of the vertebral body must be intact [49, 83, 162, 186]. KEMPF et al. [93, 94] also used compression osteosynthesis in cases where the posterior wall of the vertebral body is not intact, but can be loaded once the fracture has been reduced. The «fracture subluxation en quartier d'orange» described by him looks similar to the «rotational fracture dislocation» of HOLDSWORTH [78]. If the posterior wall of the vertebral body is not intact, the result will be unsatisfactory, as shown in Figure 18.

*Wire and spinous process plate fixation:* Fixation of the spinous processes using wire as a substitute of ruptured ligaments was the first osteosynthesis of the spine [64], and is still used in the cervical spine. KAUFER and HAYES [92] still recommended this type of fixation in the thoracic and lumbar spine as recently as 1966, but it is no longer used in isolation because of the inadequate mechanical stability. It is only occasionally used in addition to other instrumentations, because better methods are available. The same holds true for double plates applied to the spinous processes [103, 159].

*Harrington compression instrumentation* (Fig. 19). The Harrington compression instrumentation consists of a threaded rod which is shortened intraoperatively to the necessary length, with opposed hooks at either end which can be brought nearer to each other using compression nuts.

Unlike its use in scoliosis surgery where the fixation is applied to the weak transverse processes,

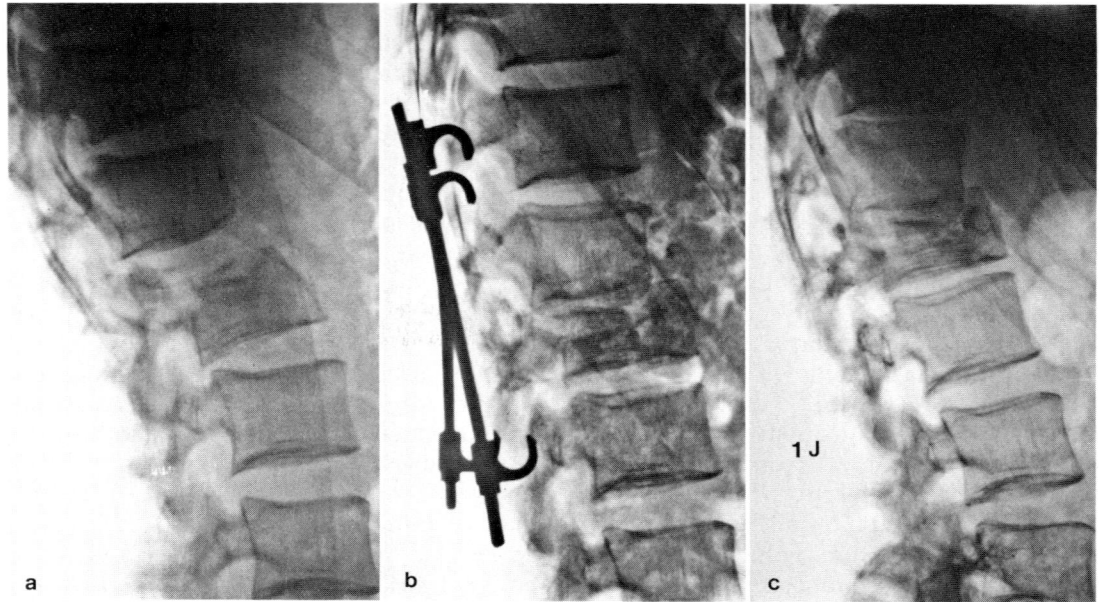

Fig. 18. L2 fracture (patient M. J. male, 22 years old) unsuitable for tension band fixation. a) The posterior third of the vertebral body is severely destroyed. The posterior wall is not suitable as fulcrum for the tension band fixation. b) under compression, the vertebra has collapsed and reduction is not possible because of this. c) one year after removal of the metal work.

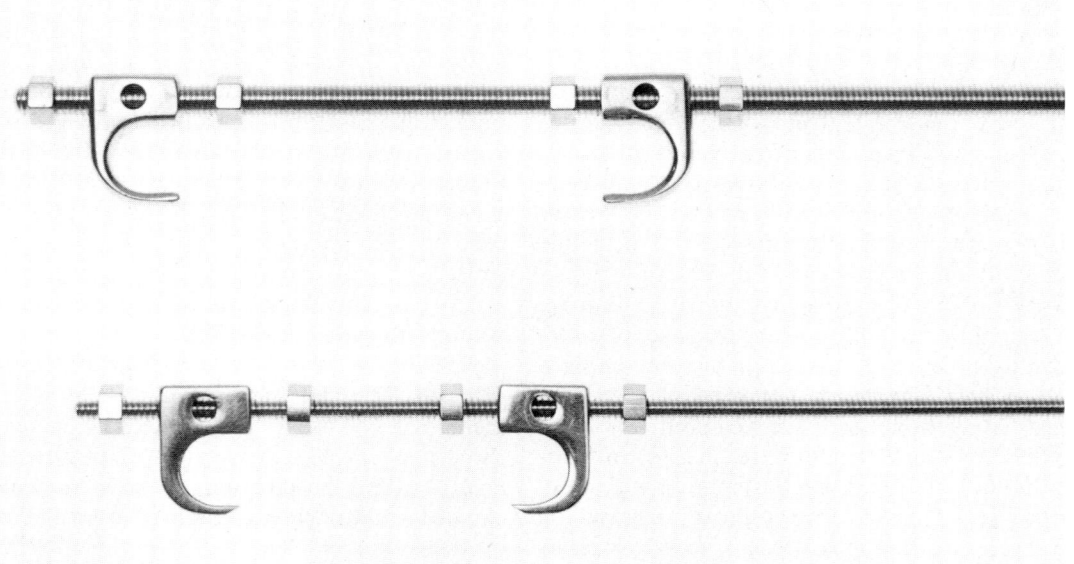

Fig. 19. Harrington compression instrumentation.

the hooks are applied underneath the laminae which provides extremely stable fixation [83]. STAUFFER and NEIL [186] found experimentally that the system collapsed by fracture of the spinal specimen elsewhere in about two thirds of the cases and by fracture of the instrumented lamina in about one third.

Using this technique, only one hook per rod needs to be placed cranially and caudally although of course both sides are instrumented. The lower hook can be placed without problems. In order not to weaken the proximal instrumented arch, for positioning of the upper hook a sufficiently large bone resection of the next higher lamina must be carried out to ensure that the hook fits properly.

If there is a purely posterior ligamentous lesion and displacement is present in a single segment, and the two adjacent arches are intact as well as the posterior wall of the vertebra, mono-segmental posterior compression instrumentation is possible. It fulfills in an almost ideal way the theoretical requirements for fracture fixation of the spine, namely the shortest fixation distance, little muscle detachment for the approach, and stability for mobilization, but unfortunately these preconditions are not frequently encountered.

Using Harrington compression in one segment, the device exerts pure traction forces. However, if the local injury pattern requires placement of the hooks on arches further apart according to WHITE et al. [209], the effect of a three-point fixation by pressure of the threaded rod on the middle arch is additionally present in the kyphotic spine. (Fig. 20).

In the original Harrington compression instrumentation, this three-point effect is not great owing to the low stiffness of the 3/16th inch threaded rod, and it does not occur in lordotic

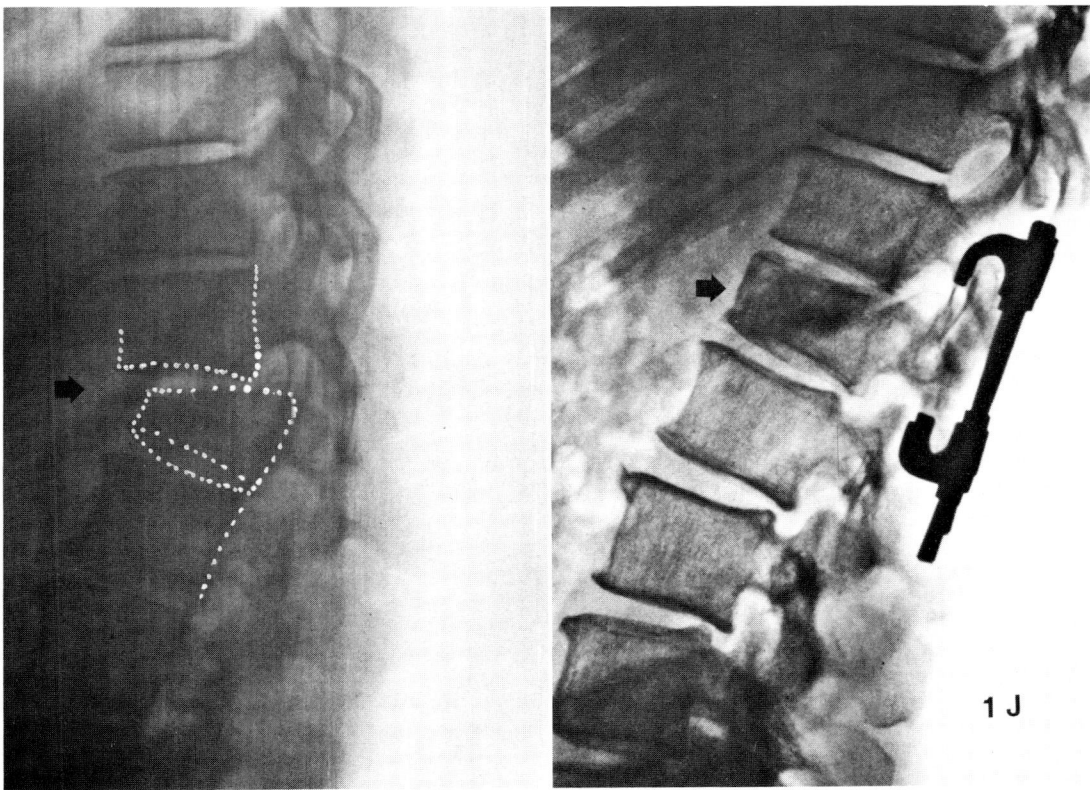

Fig. 20. Monosegmental posterior tension band fixation in a compression fracture of L1 with preserved posterior vertebral body wall, rupture of the interspinous ligaments and preserved arch of T12 and L1 (patient K.W., male, 50 years old). a) radiograph at the time of injury. b) one year postoperatively.

parts of the spine. These disadvantages are compensated for by two modifications. KEMPF et al. [93, 94] use a reversed type of distraction rod, but with the direction of the notches inverted and a reduced distance between the notches for the upper hook. The lower hook is attached in the compression mode. JACOBS et al. [82] point to the possibility of converting the locking-hook spinal rod system developed by them from a distraction system into compression system by reversal of the hooks, as described in 4.2.1.1. In this compression system, the advantages of contouring the rod into the lordosis and the rotational stabilization of the hooks are maintained. However, three to five mobile segments are bridged in this type of fixation.

The disadvantages of the Harrington compression system include the fact that reduction must be carried out first of all either by positioning of the patient or by means of a temporarily inserted distraction instrumentation in more severe rotational fracture dislocations. This instrumentation then needs to be removed. Caution is indicated where the anterior longitudinal ligament as well as the posterior ligament complex is ruptured, for example in complete dislocations or rotational fracture dislocations. In these cases, the Harrington compression as well as the distraction system will only be a type of splinting and is not a stable fixation [83, 93]. KEMPF's modification of the compression instrumentation is less stable in rotation than the ROY-CAMILLE plate [94], and no measurement data is available on rotational testing for the remaining types of compression fixation.

*Weiss springs* (Fig. 21): This dynamic, unilaterally applied instrumentation of the spine was conceived for scoliosis therapy by GRUCA [59, 60] in 1956. Strong springs are inserted overlying the laminae directly beside the spinous processes, the tension being adjustable prior to insertion. Weiss adapted the spring system for bilateral application in fracture treatment in 1965 [205, 206]. The fixation corrects kyphosis in the presence of an intact posterior vertebral body wall by the strength of the spring, which replaces the severed posterior elements in a dynamic way.

Implantation is simple [155], and the fixation takes up a small volume. Hooks which are

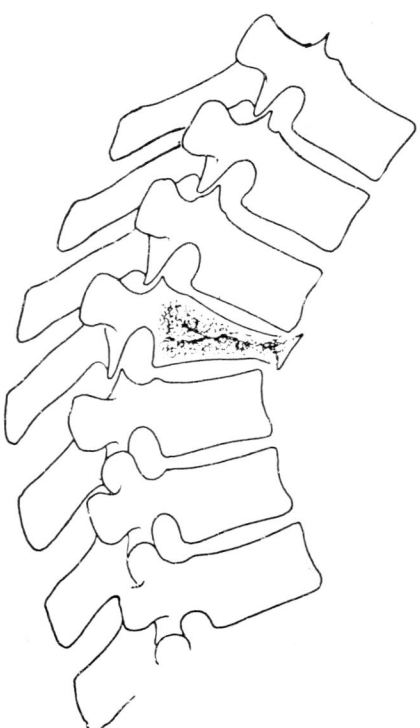
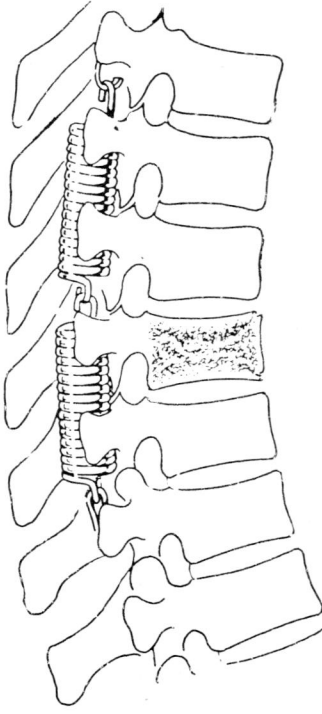

Fig. 21. Weiss spring (ref. [155]).

shaped to the anatomy of the arch and a spring loading device are available [205]. The fitting of the hooks just beside the base of the spinous processes is easy to visualize. WEISS recommends implantation in accordance with the «two vertebrae above, two vertebrae below» rule [205] and BÖTEL bridges over 3–5 segments [15, 16].

The advantages of the Weiss spring are obvious. It is the only technique where there is no iatrogenic stiffening of mobile segments of the spine (with the exception of direct osteosyntheses restricted to one vertebra, as described in section 4.1). Due to the elasticity, there is no extrusion or detachment at the anchoring points, and this has been confirmed experimentally [64, 150]. It is the only method in which mobilization can be carried out without a corset, and immediate mobilization is recommended once wound healing has occurred [15, 16, 205].

These indisputable advantages are counteracted by disadvantages which have limited wider use of the method. The stability afforded by the Weiss spring is significantly less than that which is obtained using the Harrington compression or distraction systems. It is particularly unstable in rotation. STAUFFER and NEIL saw a rotation deformity long before a flexion deformity occurred when the spine specimen was loaded in flexion and rotation. With unloading, the flexion deformity improved whereas the rotational deformity did not get better in most cases [186]. JACOBS et al. noted a kyphosis of 11.5° in pure flexion with a bending moment of 25 Nm and 19.8° at 40 Nm [83]. In addition histological investigations [205] have shown that dense fibrous tissue grows into the gaps in the spring where it is drawn apart with the tension, and this eliminates the elastic recoil of the spring. Nevertheless, it does of course still provide flexible compression with lengthening of the spring. The indications are essentially the same as those for any compression system, but are restricted in extensive damage to the vertebral arch as overcorrection may occur [16]. Particular attention should be paid to the fact that unlike the Harrington instrumentations the Weiss spring cannot be used as a splinting device in dislocations or fracture dislocations where there is complete rupture of the ventral ligaments and a three column instability, but is contraindicated in these cases.

*Tension band plating:* The tension band principle by dorsal transpedicular plating has been used by ROY-CAMILLE [163, 164, 165, 166] in appropriate cases, where there is bone in the posterior third of the vertebral bodies capable of weight bearing in association with rupture of the posterior elements. The plate acts in tension with three-point fixation, just like a compression plate used in the lateral femur after a simple femoral fracture (Fig. 22). A total of four vertebrae are included in the fixation according to ROY-CAMILLE et al. [165] (Fig. 23). JACOBS et al. have shown experimentally that the stability is equal to the Harrington compression instrumentation for flexion.

However, plate fixation using transpedicular screws is most frequently used in practice as a buttressing or neutralization plate, and is discussed in section 4.2.1.3.

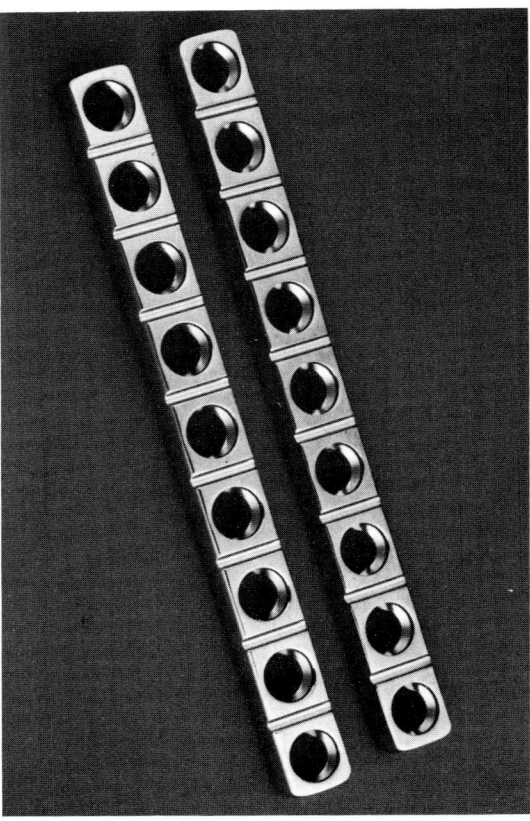

Fig. 22. Modified spinal plate described by ROY-CAMILLE (AO-ASIF).

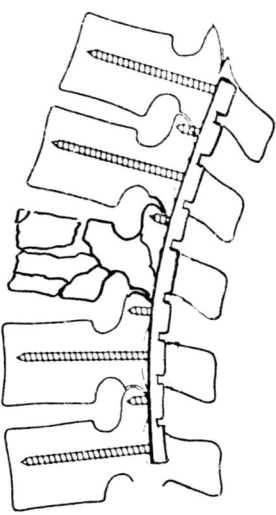

Fig. 23. Diagram of correctly placed Roy-Camille plate.

*External fixator:* The external fixator can be used just as well in compression as in distraction in the appropriate fracture situation, and acts by dorsal compression. The observation under 4.2.1.1. remains valid.

### 4.2.1.3 *Buttressing techniques using multipoint fixation*

Analysis of the biomechanical action of Harrington distraction instrumentation (4.2.1.1) demonstrates that besides the distraction effect, the reduction of kyphosis and stability against flexion are both achieved by three-point fixation where the vertebral arch is not fractured, or by four-point fixation to the adjacent arches where the lamina is fractured. It is possible to resort completely to multi-point fixation and to dispense with distraction provided:

a) a distraction force is not necessary for secure anchoring of the implant on the spine as with the Harrington distraction rod, and

b) distraction of the fragments with the implant is not necessary, where the posterior wall of the fractured vertebra is intact or has already been restored either by positioning of the patient or by open reduction.

Precondition a) is present in implants which are not inserted with hooks on the lamina, but which have firm fixation with the bone, for example where screws are firmly fixed in a pedicle (Roy-Camille plates and their modifications), or where wire loops completely surround the lamina (LUQUE).

Precondition b) may be attained by temporary insertion of a distraction rod or an outrigger for reduction, even if open reduction and manual leverage on the spinous and articular processes have not been successful in very severe fracture dislocations as in Figure 1.

*Neutralization plate:* In contrast to the earlier plates applied to the spinous processes [76, 212], osteosynthesis using a dorsal plate with transpedicular screws (introduced by ROY-CAMILLE in 1963) attains its stability from pull-out resistant screws firmly fixed in the pedicles and vertebral bodies and by its direct support on the facet joints. It thus neutralizes forces acting on the spine [163, 164, 165, 166]. In order to be able to pass the screws through the pedicles into the vertebral bodies, ROY-CAMILLE chose half the normal distance between the pedicles at the thoracolumbar region (26 mm) as the distance between the holes in the plate, i.e. 13 mm. Thus the intermediate holes between the screws passing into the pedicles are located over the articular processes, providing good purchase for additional screws. The very stiff, 1 cm wide plates are precontoured to the normal shape of the spine and can be further contoured during the operation with bending pliers. In order to avoid a reduction in stability and danger of fracturing of the plate at the screw holes, the plates are reinforced in thickness at the level of each hole. There exist some plate modifications with slight variations in thickness (Teinturier, AO-ASIF).

The operation is technically difficult because a direct view of the pedicles is not possible via the posterior approach. The point of entry for the screw must hence be determined with the knowledge of the normal anatomy of each vertebra, modified according to the radiographs of the individual vertebra. This requires experience in spinal surgery with good three-dimensional conceptualization. Exact instructions are available from LOUIS [107], ROY-CAMILLE et al. [163, 164, 165, 166] and SAILLANT [170]. The transverse processes and the intervertebral joints serve as reference points.

Not only the point of entry, but also the direction of the screws is critical. Too much convergence may lead to penetration into the vertebral canal. Divergence may lead to penetration of the screw outside the vertebral body. ROY-CAMILLE recommends a 45 mm screw length for the lumbar region and 35 mm for the thoracic region [165]. He warns that it is senseless and dangerous to introduce the screws as far as the anterior margin of the vertebral body. Screws anchored in the articular processes should have a length of at most 15–19 mm. They should not penetrate the opposite cortex in order to avoid injuring the nerve root lying below. In order to ensure that the plate acts as a neutralization plate, the fixation must include two intact vertebrae above and below the fracture. As a rule, five vertebrae are thus included in the fixation. This fixation distance is shortened by one vertebra only in pure or almost pure dislocations since compression is mainly carried out here [165].

The advantages of transpedicular plate fixation are substantial:

- Great stability is attained due to fixation of the articular processes and the vertebral arch. WÖRSDÖRFER found this to be the most stable form of fixation. With a bending moment of 10 Nm, there is a flexion deformation of 1.4° in the injured area as compared with 2.2° at 15 Nm. Loosening of the screws and plastic deformation of the plate only occurred at 40 Nm [214]. KEMPF et al. [94] found the plate fixation more stable than the Harrington instrumentation, and found stability to be comparable with that of the uninjured spine, particularly in rotation.
- Plates fixed with transpedicular screws acting as neutralization plates can be used in any type of fracture whether or not there is damage to the ligaments, or to the posterior wall of the vertebral body. In comminuted vertebral body fractures, collapse in craniocaudal direction is prevented by the fixed distance between the plate holes and kyphosis by the stiffness of the plate and the tensile strength of the screws. Using a neutralization plate, the initial biomechanical situation of the fracture type does not play such a crucial role as in other fixation systems, provided that the reduction has been successful.
- Due to the shape of the plates, the physiological curvature of the spine with a lumbar lordosis can be restored in an optimal way.

As against these advantages, there are also the following disadvantages:

- Plate fixation is not only stable, but also very rigid. In contrast to long bones, high bending, shear and tensile loads and movements occur at the necks of the screws at the ends of the plate, due to the mobility between spinal segments. These stresses and movements lead to increased screw breakages after a few weeks or months (e.g. in 17 out of 44 patients reported by ROY-CAMILLE et al. [165]). For this reason, MUHR and TSCHERNE [138] recommended a second anterior procedure in major anterior defects.
- The distance between the holes of the Roy-Camille plate are suited to the average anatomy. However the holes are not always appropriately sited to suit the distance between the pedicles in each individual case. Occasionally oblique placement of the screws may be helpful and is often possible due to the width of the pedicles [165], or plate modifications such as slit hole plates may be used.
- Fixation of the plate sometimes requires partial flattening of facet joints using an osteotome. In other cases, the joint is damaged by the intra-articular screw, or the capsule is damaged by the pressure of the plate, so that mobility remains restricted over the entire length of the plate, even after plate removal. Dispensing with screw fixation of the plate at the articular processes entails up to a 50% loss of stability (WÖRSDÖRFER [214]).
- Classically, the dorsal plate requires incorporation of two vertebrae above and two vertebrae below the fracture, thus leading to fixation of four motion segments. However, ROY-CAMILLE [167] recently developed a modification for the lumbar spine allowing the pedicles of the two terminal vertebrae to be gripped with two screws. Thus the fixation distance can be restricted to three vertebrae (two motion segments), even using the plate. This eliminates the most important disadvantage of this type of fixation.
- The broad plate which is apposed to the arches and facet joints reduces the space available for bony fusion [214].
- As has already been mentioned, the operative technique is difficult, and its practical use is thus restricted to surgeons who are constantly practicing spinal surgery in all its forms.

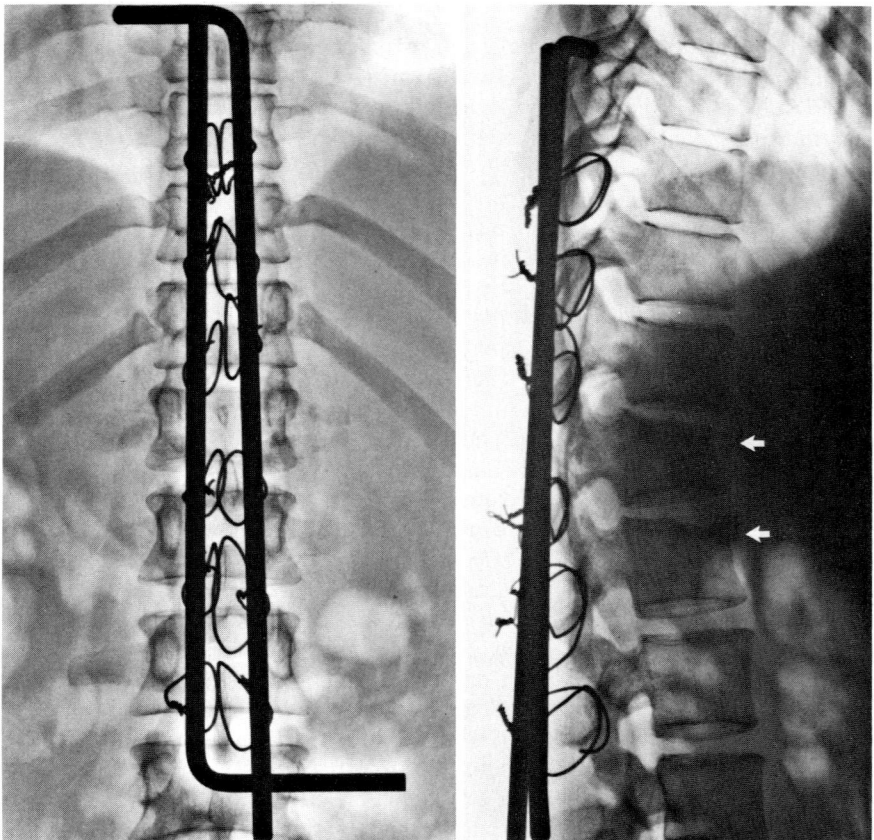

Fig. 24. Segmental sublaminar instrumentation described by Luque [109] (patient P.A., female, 27 years old).

– Reduction of the fracture itself is not possible with the plate and must be achieved beforehand. Correction of displacement in the AP plane can be achieved by positioning and movement of the patient on the operation table, and Roy-Camille et al. [165] recommend use of an orthopaedic table. Compression fractures or locked dislocations can be reduced either by manipulation or by temporary insertion of an outrigger or Harrington distraction rod prior to plate fixation.

*Luque segmental sublaminar instrumentation* (Fig. 24). This method of fixation was developed by Luque [109, 110, 111] for correction of scoliosis. All the instrumented vertebrae are closely bound to the longitudinal rod by sublaminar wires bilaterally giving multi-point fixation. The wire loops take up the traction forces. The strong longitudinal rods which are smooth-surfaced and shaped to the physiological curve of the spine take up the forces applied to the vertebral arch. Rotation of the rods, which would transform a lumbar lordosis into a kyphosis, can be prevented by bending the end of the rod through a right angle (Fig. 24). The transverse part can also be anchored in the pelvis as necessary.

This implant has become well known in scoliosis surgery because mobilization is possible without any external support. This great stability has led to its use recently in fracture treatment [1, 111, 124]. Ferguson et al. [48] reported 54 thoracolumbar fractures in 1983, which were treated with this technique without external postoperative support.

The implant, which was originally developed for use with intact vertebral bodies, does not provide any stability in the axial direction because the wires slide along the rods, although its stability is otherwise very good [207]. It thus cannot prevent healing of a burst fracture with some vertebral collapse, when the posterior wall of the vertebra or dorsal structures are damaged. Thus the indications for this type of fixation are very restricted, especially since the fixation must involve many vertebral segments. FERGUSON [48] anchored the rods as far away as the pelvis in some cases. Indeed, LUQUE et al. [111] regard this as essential in all paraplegic patients. In reducing vertebrae, they recommend the use of an outrigger, and the use of C-shaped rods bent to right angles on both ends, which maintain distraction by support on the spinous processes. Using Luque rods without anchoring at the pelvis can allow rod rotation as reported by WENGER et al. [207], although these authors describe sophisticated techniques for wiring the ends of the rods.

### 4.2.1.4 Neutralization techniques without multipoint support on the arches

*External fixator:* All other systems mentioned so far have in common a mobile connection between the anchoring point in the vertebra and the longitudinal support, whether this is a hook against the vertebral arch, a screw against the plate hole or a wire loop against the rod. Therefore, besides the anchoring site, a further bony support is necessary for fixation of the spine: in four-point bending systems these are the arches of the adjacent vertebrae, and in tension banding systems they are the posterior edges of the vertebral bodies.

The external fixator is the only system in which the instrumented vertebra is fixed in three dimensions by the device itself: the transpedicular screws do not allow any mobility between the bone and the implant, and the screws are in turn fixed firmly in all directions by the fixator frame. Thus, a further bony support is not necessary biomechanically, and the instrumentation can be restricted to the two vertebrae directly adjacent to the fracture, even when a burst fracture is present with destroyed posterior wall of the vertebral body. For the same reason, this system can also serve simply to neutralize damaging forces and to maintain the reduction already attained by patient positioning or manipulation of the

Schanz screws even without a distraction or compression effect.

### 4.2.1.5 Combined techniques

It is logical to use a combination of various procedures in an attempt to reduce the disadvantages which may occur with individual techniques. Combining Harrington distraction instrumentation with segmental sublaminar wiring as described by Luque leads to an appreciable increase in stability. It also reduces the danger of hook dislocation [2, 52, 53, 101, 189], but hook dislocations still have been reported [1, 74]. GAINES et al. [52] has shown experimentally an increase of 25–60% in the stability of the fixation as compared with simple Harrington rod fixation. The greatest percentage increase in stability was in rotation, rotational stability being still very poor.

WENGER et al. [207] demonstrated a similar increase in stability for axial and flexion stresses in the experimental situation. Clinically, this combination has proved effective for scoliosis surgery (Fig. 25) in the vast majority of our cases, and makes followup treatment simpler and safer [57, 74].

However, segmental instrumentation does not completely prevent hook dislocation, as demonstrated in Figure 26. A lordotically bent Harrington rod can rotate into kyphosis as reported by SULLIVAN et al. [189] in spite of the sublaminar wiring, and the only way of preventing rotation is to use square ended rods or the locking hook spinal rod system.

There are several reports of the combination of Harrington distraction instrumentation with Harrington compression instrumentation for individual cases where there is a scoliotic curve secondary to a fracture, or for improvement of stability [56, 106, 174, 182, 190]. However, these reports amount only to a very small fraction of the reported series. The combination is rarely necessary since lateral deviation can usually be corrected without this combination. Another combination described by BÖTEL [15, 16] is interesting biomechanically. Where there is a fracture with destruction of the posterior wall of the vertebral body, he superimposes a short plate with transpedicular screws or a short Knodt distraction rod with the longer Weiss spring.

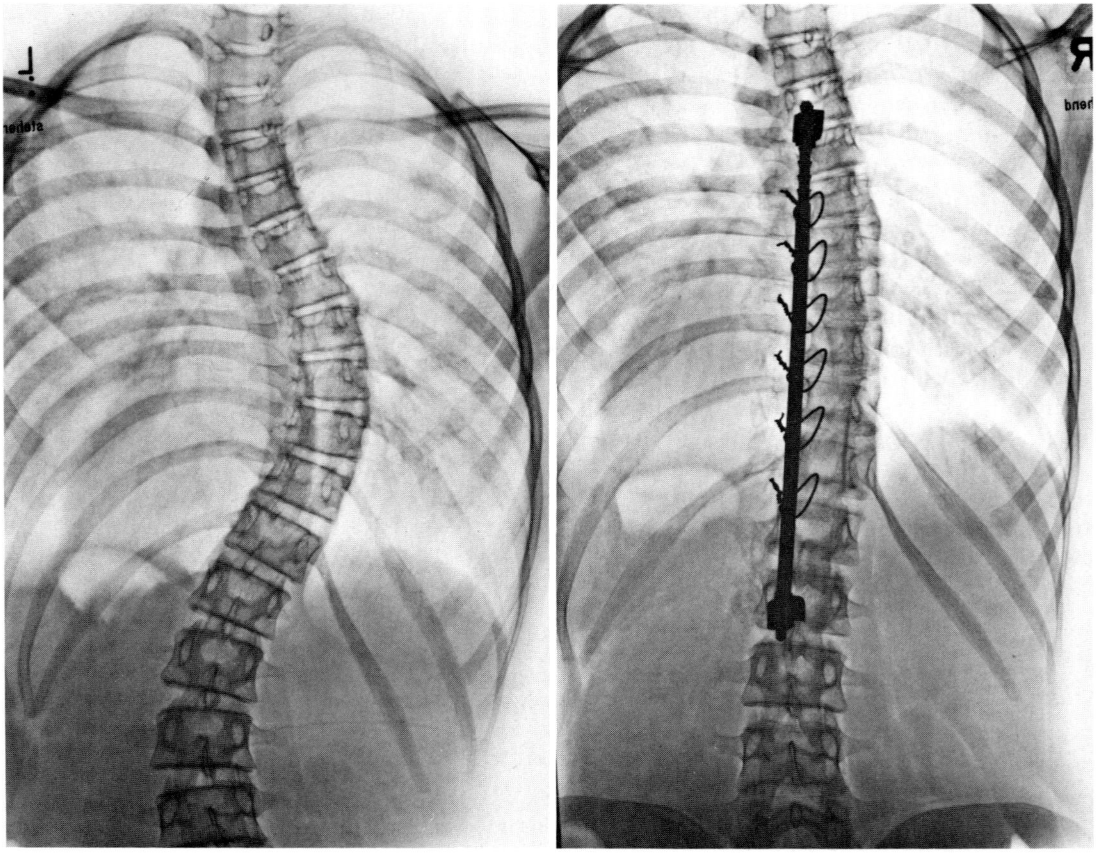

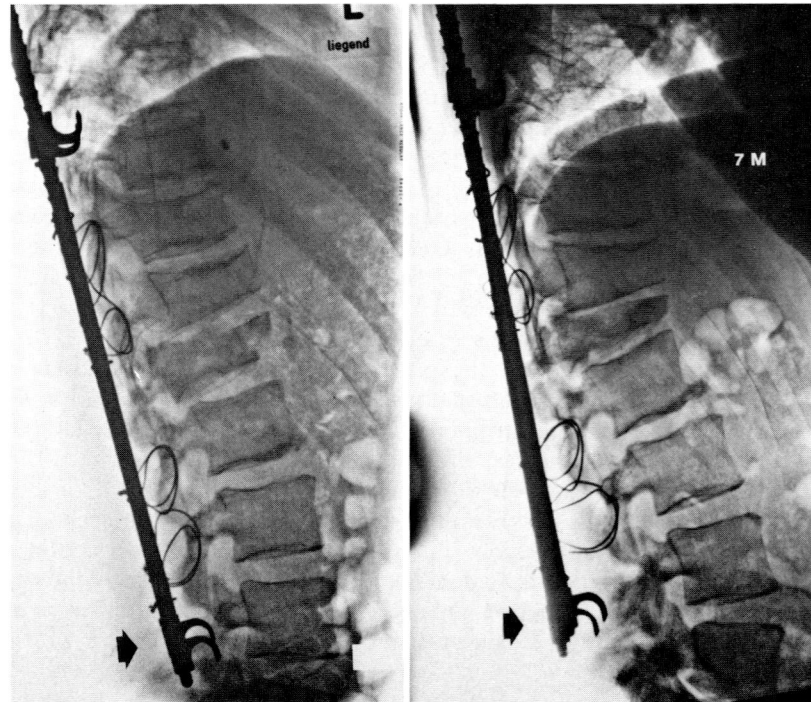

Fig. 26. Dislocation of the lower Harrington hooks despite segmental sublaminar wiring and «three vertebrae above, three vertebrae below» technique (patient B.H., male, 29 years old, seven months post operation).

Thus the fixation distance can be kept very short with a rigid implant, because this only has to stabilize the vertebrae adjacent ot the fracture. The kyphosing forces are counteracted by the flexible spring compression fixation. This in turn reduces the flexion stress on the plate and screws and protects them from fatigue fracture [16].

WEBER and MAGERL [204] recommended combined tension band wires and bone cement for occasional use as temporary fixation until definitive surgery was possible. OPPEL and BROCK [145] recommend a combination of multilayer Dacron gauze and bone cement [146]. Both techniques depend entirely on the spinous processes being stable and viable and are no longer indicated in thoracolumbar fractures.

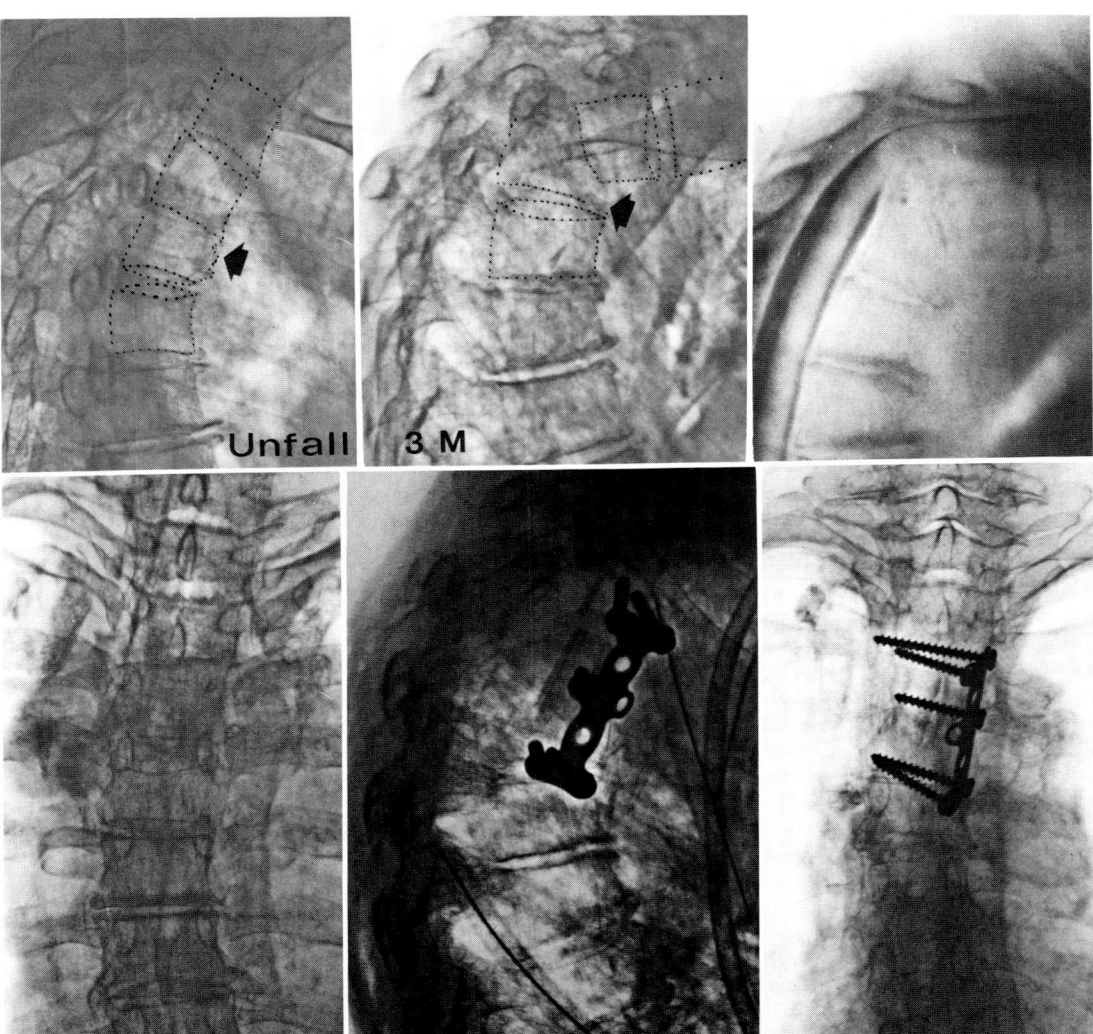

Fig. 27. Fracture of T4 with secondary increase in kyphosis. Three months after injury, the first neurological signs occur. Thoracotomy with anterior decompression, reduction, bone grafting and Orozco plate. Regression of all symptoms (patient S. B., female, 68 years old).

### 4.2.2 Anterior techniques

Surgical techniques of anterior spinal decompression with subsequent bone grafting will be dealt with in section 4.3. However, the immediate stability of the bone graft may be improved using fixation anteriorly through the same approach, in order to shorten the period of postoperative immobilization. The fixation has two functions, first to prevent displacement of the graft and secondly to weight bear until the bone graft has healed.

#### 4.2.2.1 *Anterior plate fixation*

Special plates for fixation of the anterior vertebral bodies following bone grafting from the anterior approach in the thoracic and lumbar region do not so far exist. For this reason, implants available in other fields of traumatology are used. In the upper thoracic spine, triple H plates as described by OROZCO and LLOVET [147] are most suitable because of the shape and dimensions. This fixation requires little space and has proved very effective in the cervical spine.

The new cervical spine double slit plate described by CASPAR [26] is also suitable. Both plates have the primary function of holding the bone graft in place. However, their use in the thoracic spine is rarely indicated [38].

In the lower thoracic and the lumbar spine, the anatomy allows the use of conventional plates used in fractures of the lower limbs. These are anchored in the vertebral bodies adjacent to the fractured vertebra. All the vertebral discs which are bridged by the fixation must be included in the fusion, otherwise screw breakage or loosening of the screws is unavoidable.

One advantage of the system is that two motion segments less are fused than when using posterior distraction systems or posterior plates. Another advantage is the possibility of anterior spinal decompression by excision of the vertebral body. However, fixation with anterior plates has the following disadvantages:
- Due to the surgical approach and the anatomy in the lumbar region, the plate is not applied anteriorly but anterolaterally to one or other side, whereas in the cervical spine it is applied

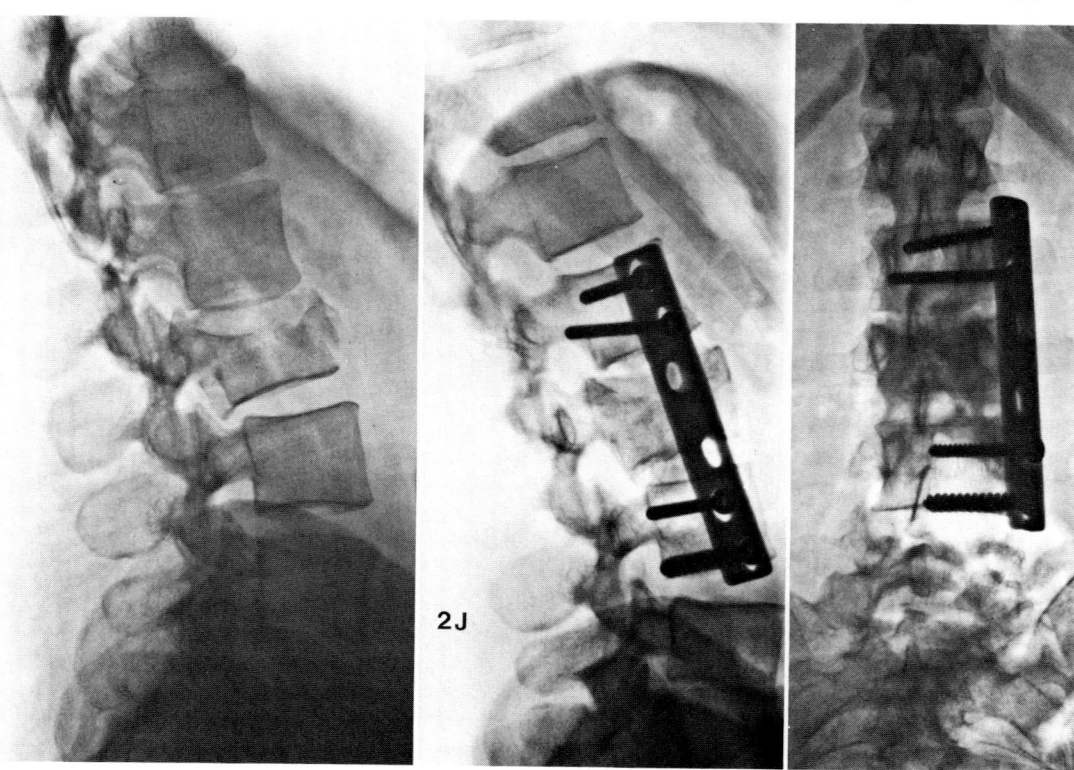

Fig. 28. Example of anterior plate fixation in L3 fracture (O.R., female, 34 years old).

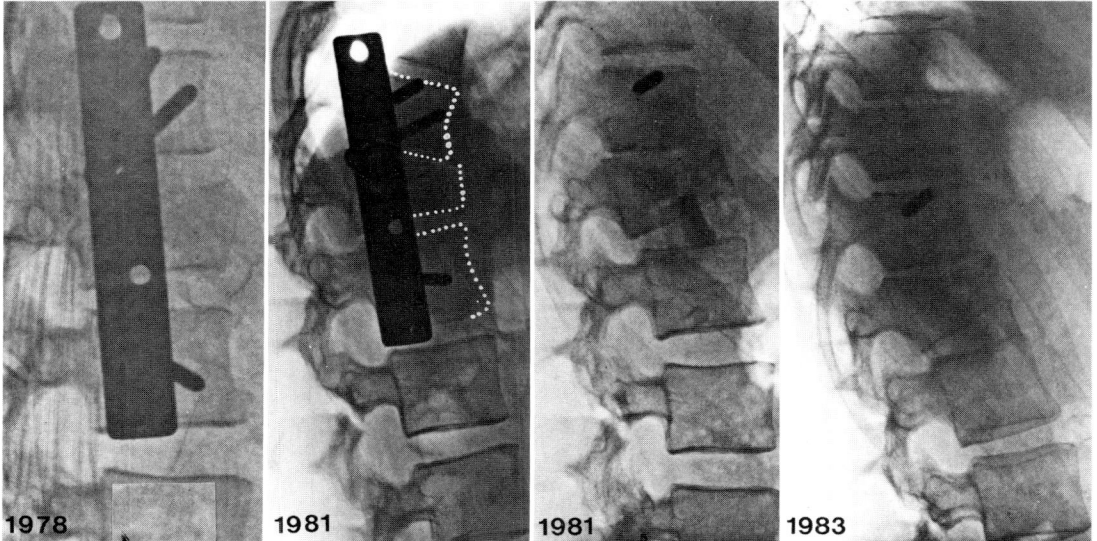

**Fig. 29a.** Situation after anterior plate fixation of an L1 fracture with recurrence of kyphosis and screw breakage. Further anterior surgery with plate removal, corrective osteotomy L1/2 and intercorporeal bone grafting (patient E.S., female, 27 years old). Note the plate which is too long cranially.

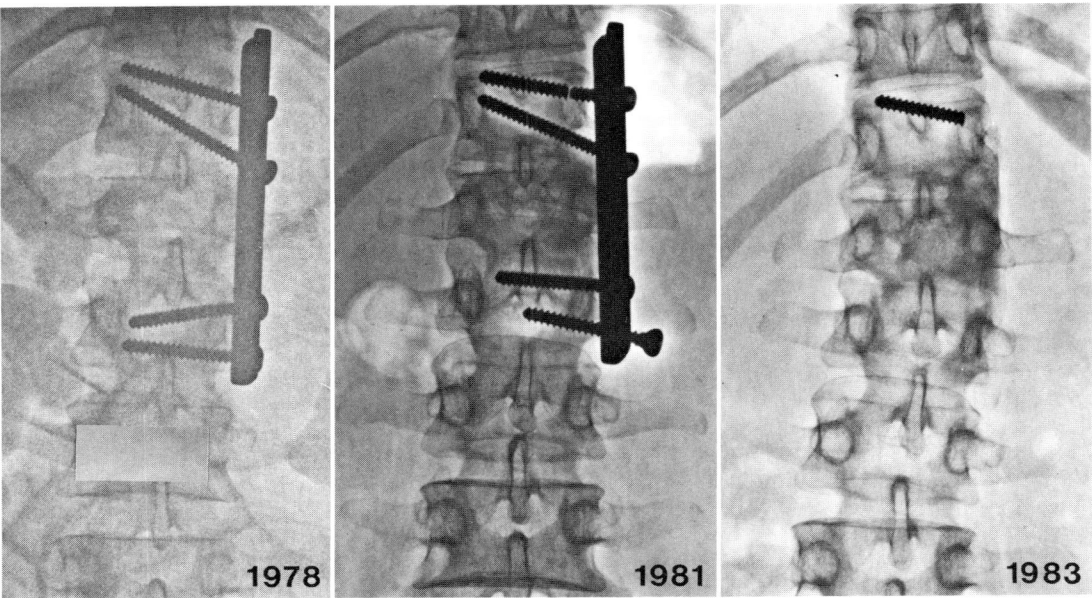

**Fig. 29b.** AP radiograph of the same patient.

anteriorly. If there is no adequate bony support on the opposite side, there is danger of scoliotic deviation in the area of the fracture with flexion.

– The length of the plates and the positioning of the holes in the plates are often unsuitable. In order to accomodate two screws in the cranial and caudal terminal vertebrae, these screw holes often have to be drilled very obliquely. In addition, the projecting end of the plate may come in contact with the neighboring vertebra beyond the intervertebral disc which can lead to loosening (Fig. 29).

– The neck of the screws tend to cut through the

41

thin lateral vertebral cortex. The lateral screw reinforcement clips enclosing the vertebral bodies in anterior scoliosis instrumentation according to DWYER [47] and ZIELKE [220, 221] cannot be used to prevent this complication. The fixation is probably not stable enough to allow early mobilization, particularly when there is dorsal bony or ligamentous injury. There is little experimental data available, and only JACOBS et al. [83] have investigated a «Boehler plate» for pure ventral vertebral injuries. They found low stability with 20° kyphosis at 20 Nm flexion stress. Attempts to pull out the screw perpendicular to the vertebral surface showed high pull-out forces with cancellous screws when compared to cortical screws [192], but these experiments do not reproduce the direction of forces which occur in vivo.

– Revision surgery in implant displacements or implant removal are very much more difficult and risky than in dorsal procedures because of scarring which occurs with this approach.

### 4.2.2.2 Anterior rod fixation

Instead of anterior plates, it has been suggested that the VDS fixation described by ZIELKE for scoliosis surgery should be used to secure a massive intercorporeal bone graft which absorbs compression forces. The threaded rod is fixed to the vertebral bodies with screws [195] in the compression mode, thus locking the graft. Using the same VDS screws, SLOT [181] uses a thicker rod with a thread at the ends only, which can be used for distraction and thus for direct correction of the kyphosis. Anchoring of the VDS screws in the vertebral bodies can be enhanced by clips.

In 1984, various anterior rod systems were presented independently by DUNN [45], KANEDA [91] and KOSTUIK [99]. These systems attempt to attain a better stability with double rods. They have two important advantages:

1. Complete anterior decompression is possible by resection of the posterior wall of the vertebral body.
2. The fixation remains restricted to three vertebrae, but any intervertebral disc which is bridged over must be included in the fusion. Occasionally unisegmental fixation and fusion between two vertebrae are possible in certain types of fracture.

The following disadvantages of anterior instrumentation should be mentioned:

– In the emergency situation, the anterior thoracolumbar approach requires greater surgical skill.
– If complications occur, re-operation is more difficult due to scar formation. Routine removal of metal after healing is thus not advisable.
– Most dural injuries are situated posteriorly and cannot be dealt with surgically from the anterior approach.
– The stability of anterior instrumentation without additional posterior stabilization is not adequate for immediate mobilization without a plaster jacket.
– Where there is a combined anterior and posterior injury, adequate correction of the kyphosis without late recurrence is rarely successful using anterior instrumentation only because the dorsal tension banding structures are severed and tend to separate under flexion forces. Thus usually additional compression instrumentation would be necessary posteriorly to improve the reduction and stability.
– Large anterior implants may lead to secondary vascular injury.

## 4.3 Bone grafts

### 4.3.1 Intercorporeal bone grafts through the anterior approach

As mentioned in Section 3.2, laminectomy is not a suitable method of decompression in thoracic and lumbar fractures, except in cases where parts of the vertebral arch are penetrating the vertebral canal. Spinal cord or cauda equina compression is mostly anterior, arising from the posterior edge of the vertebral body, from kyphotic deformity and from displacement of posterior wall fragments or of intervertebral disc material. Thus removal of the arch does not lead to decompression but only to increased instability, that can cause an increase in neural compression due to the increase in kyphosis [27, 122]. The only indications for laminectomy are for removal of debris, repair of dural tears or impaction of posterior wall fragments back into the vertebral body, when fracture reduction did not restore adequate cross-sectional width of the spinal canal. However, even as a surgical approach route to supplementary measures laminectomy is of limited usefulness, since undesired manipulation of the swollen neural tissue cannot be avoided.

Standardized surgical approaches make it possible to decompress all regions of the spine at the site of the pathology [107, 134, 196]. Anterior decompression by partial resection of the vertebral body and its posterior wall allows exposure of the dura by partial vertebrectomy, and enables it to be freed from any anterior structures which may be compressing the dura.

Computer tomography of the injured spine is useful because better analysis of the fractures is possible as well as improving the diagnosis of canal compression by bone or intervertebral disc (Fig. 30). These are seen better than on a plain radiograph [21, 46, 55, 124, 210], whereas the latter shows a kyphotic deformity better.

Computerized tomography gives exact information on the size and localization of fragments displaced into the vertebral canal, especially when software is available to reassemble the cuts longitudinally. It provides information as to whether anterior or posterior decompression is required. LINDAHL et al. [104] have shown that cortical bone splinters of a thickness of 0.6 mm and cancellous bone fragments from 1.2 mm will be shown. It should be pointed out that only massive narrowing of the cross-section of the spinal canal which is not corrected by fracture reduction, requires additional surgical mea-

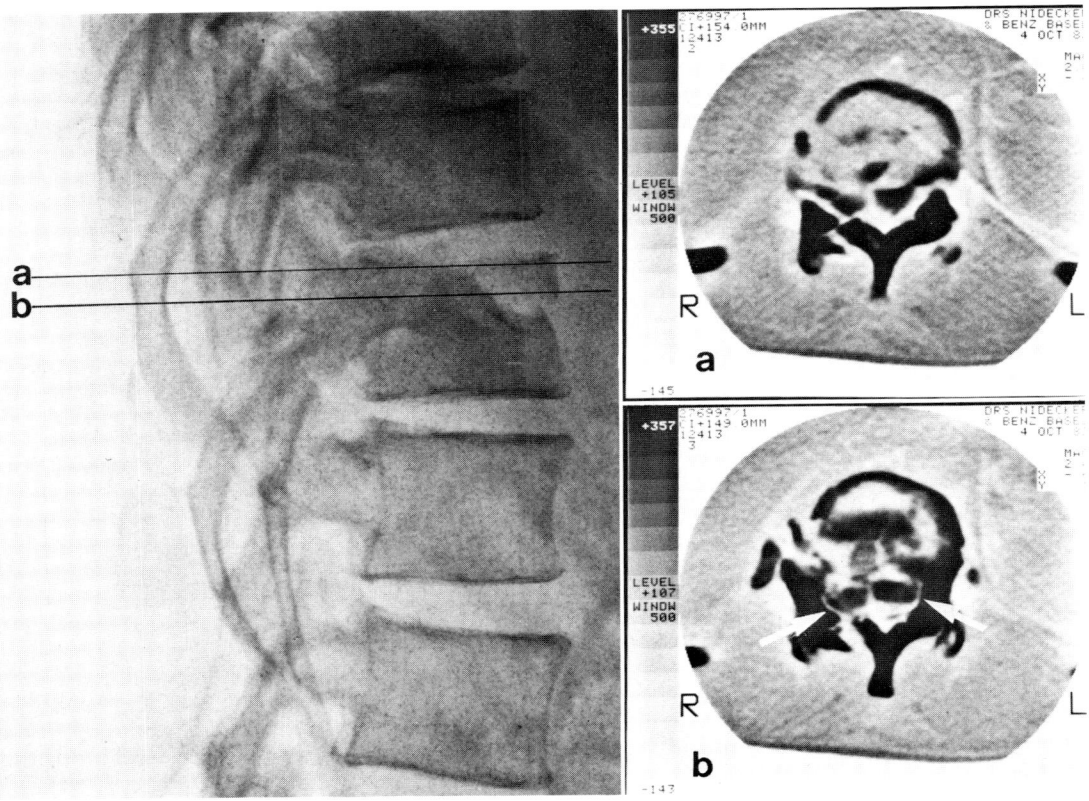

Fig. 30. Shown in the plain radiograph on the left, T12 fracture appears to be well reduced. However, subsequent computerized tomogram sections a and b show a massive reduction of the cross-sectional area of the vertebral canal, due to comminution of the posterior vertebral wall (patient A.B., male, 27 years old).

sures. Removal of small epidural or intradural splinters is not indicated, since exploring for these splinters does more harm than good.

Having performed an anterior surgical decompression, it is necessary to bridge the defect with cortical bone inserted between the cranial and caudal vertebrae to correct the deformity and to stabilize the spine by intercorporeal fusion [44, 130, 134, 150, 156, 218].

Before ossification of the intercorporeal fusion mass has taken place, the bone graft area has low stability, especially in the presence of ligamentous lesions. YOUNG et al. [218], and MOON et al. [127], hence recommend that the patients should be kept recumbent for three months postoperatively. Despite this, extrusion of the graft, collapse or sinking into the anchoring vertebrae may occur [18], with the result that anterior bone grafting is most commonly combined with some type of internal fixation as described by DUNN [45], KANEDA [91], KOSTUIK [99] or ZIELKE [220] as described in section 4.2.2.2. RISKA and MYLLYNEN [157] suggest additional fixation dorsally with Harrington instrumentation.

However, where there is a pure vertebral body compression fracture with preserved posterior body wall and intact ligaments, anterior bone grafting without additional fixation has an established place. This is because the cortical bone graft is only applied unisegmentally, and can be anchored firmly against the tight ligamentous apparatus. Cancellous bone is used to fill the remaining space in the defect, and the intervertebral disc space.

The indications for surgical treatment in this type of compression fracture, where neurological complications are rare, are discussed in Section 3.1. These fractures can usually be reduced well by lordosis, although an anterior defect is then left. According to MORSCHER [134], surgery should be considered where the anterior wall of the vertebral body is reduced to less than 50% of its normal height. MACNAB [112] suggested that if this occurs, a painful condition will result due to incongruence of the intervertebral joints. Surgery should be considered also in patients with a poor capacity to compensate for a resulting kyphosis due to pre-existing kyphotic deformities or a stiff spine, in younger patients and in patients involved in particularly strenuous occupations. This is not an emergency procedure and is best carried out 10 days after the injury

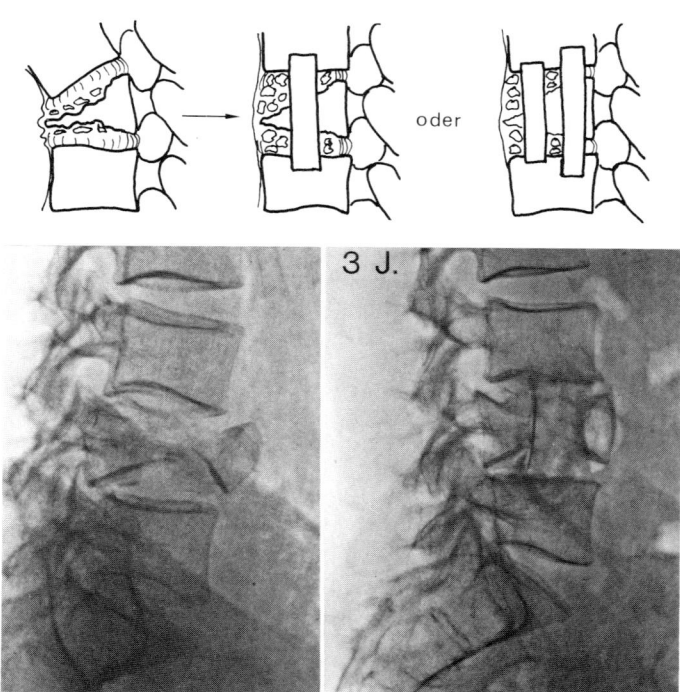

Fig. 31. L4 fracture, intercorporeal fusion L3–5. (patient H.K., male, 58 years old).

after resolution of the hematoma and the tendency to bleed. The approach is made extrapleurally and retroperitoneally at the thoracolumbar junction through the bed of the excised left 12th rib, as described by MORSCHER [134] (Fig. 32). In the lumbar spine, the retroperitoneal approach through the flank is the same as that used for a symphathectomy.

### 4.3.2 Corrective osteotomies

Bone grafting can only be applied in fresh compression fractures, whereas spinal osteotomy is necessary in late deformity [95, 134]. It is indicated where a fracture has healed with pronounced wedging and the deformity is symptomatic. The osteotomy is made through one of the two adjacent discs which is resected (see Figs. 5 and 29).

The kyphosis is then corrected manually by pressure on the spinous processes from posteriorly. The intervertebral space is widened anteriorly using a powerful vertebral spreader, and a broad load-resistant cortical graft of either autologous or homologous bone is driven in, which holds the kyphosis in the corrected position. The remaining intervertebral space is tightly filled with cancellous bone. MALCOLM regards additional posterior fixation as necessary [122], whereas MORSCHER did not report any pseudarthroses in his cases treated without fixation [129, 130, 134]. An advantage of anterior intercorporeal bone grafting is the short fusion, with correction at the site of the lesion. Disadvantages include a major operation with the anterior approach at the thoracolumbar junction, poor primary stability in isolated bone grafts and the danger of collapse.

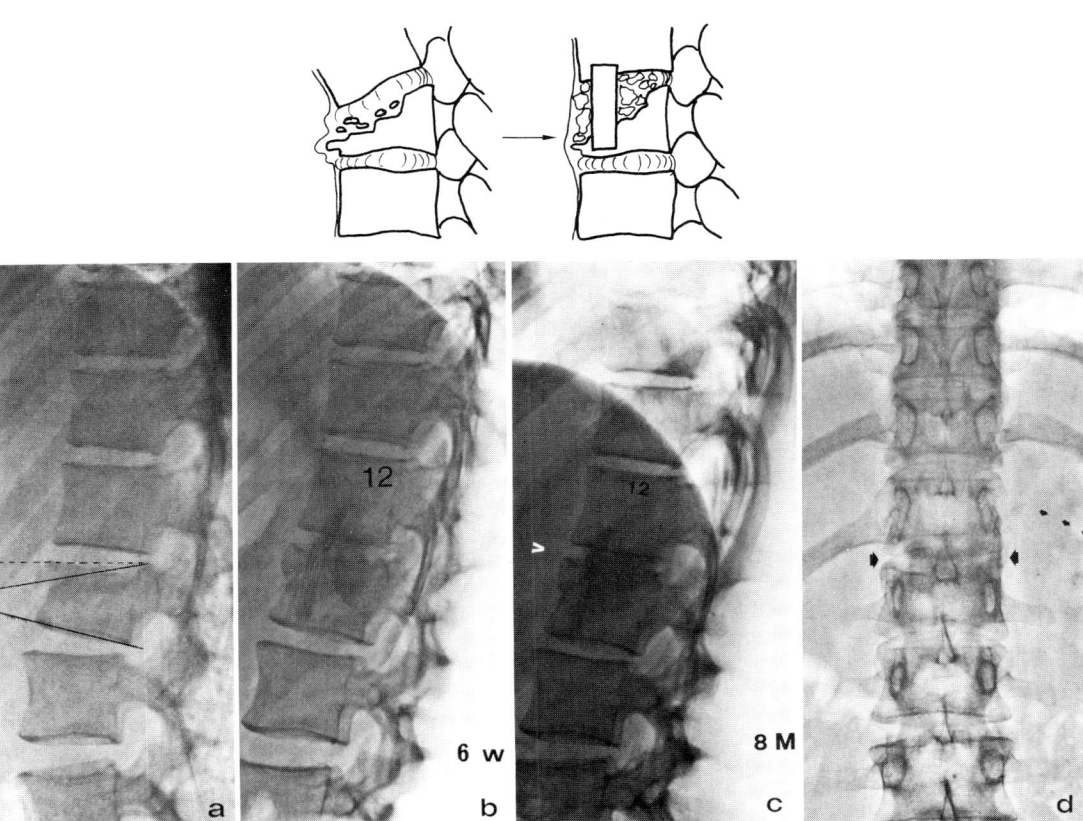

Fig. 32. Pure L 1 compression fracture with intact ligamentous structures posteriorly. a) radiograph after postural reduction for 48 hours (broken line). The posttraumatic wedge shape is shown on the solid line. b) monosegmental intercorporeal bone graft. c) no loss of correction after 8 months. d) the AP radiograph shows the resection of the 12th rib on the left for the approach as described by MORSCHER [134].

45

### 4.3.3 Transpedicular cancellous bone grafting

In fractures of the tibial plateau the bony defect which has arisen as a result of the injury is filled with cancellous bone through a cortical window. The same principle can be used in vertebral compression fractures, using the pedicle as a window. Through a posterior approach the pedicle of the fractured vertebra is drilled as if to apply a pedicular screw, but with a thicker drill bit (up to 6 mm). A slightly bent impactor can then be introduced into the vertebral body through the pedicle and the cancellous bone within the vertebra is pressed against the end plates and against the anterior wall of the vertebra so that a central cavity is formed. This is then tightly filled with small fragments of impacted cancellous bone graft. This requires an enormous amount of cancellous bone graft before the vertebra is filled. The method is described in more detail in Section 8.2.

DANIAUX [31, 32] described the technique and clinical results of transpedicular cancellous bone grafting in 1982. He combines this with screw fixation of the facet joints to the vertebra above.

Of course the deformity must be corrected pre-operatively, and the posterior wall of the vertebral body must be intact. A plaster jacket or full contact corset is required as additional fixation for three or four months post-operatively.

### 4.3.4 Additional fusions combined with instrumentation of vertebral fractures

Most authors carry out a posterior or posterolateral fusion in addition to instrumentation of a vertebral fracture. This is intended to replace the implant once the bone graft has consolidated [43, 46, 49, 56, 81, 114, 115, 148, 162, 200, 217]. The extent of the bone graft is frequently not specified in detail, but DICKSON et al. [43] used the entire instrumented distance in complete paraplegia and the region of the fracture only in partial paraplegia. SOREFF et al. [182] and JACOBS et al. [8] considered it important that only the vertebrae immediately proximal and distal to the fracture were included in the fusion mass, particularly since JACOBS et al. applied distraction rods according to the rule «three vertebrae above, three vertebrae below» (long rod – short fusion).

KEMPF et al. [93] and ARMSTRONG and JOHNSTON [6] on the other hand argue that the spine becomes stable once the fracture has consolidated except in purely ligamentous lesions and do not use a fusion.

In Weiss spring instrumentations, fusion is not used due to its mechanism of action.

Every rigid implant applied to the mobile vertebral column is in danger of fatigue fracture, even long after the fracture has become consolidated and is capable of carrying loads. An implant which is longer than the region of the bony fusion thus requires removal, in contrast to instrumentation in scoliosis where the fusion is applied over the entire length of the implant. Nine to 12 months after surgery is probably a suitable time for removal of metal work, the risk of implant failure increasing after this time [81, 84].

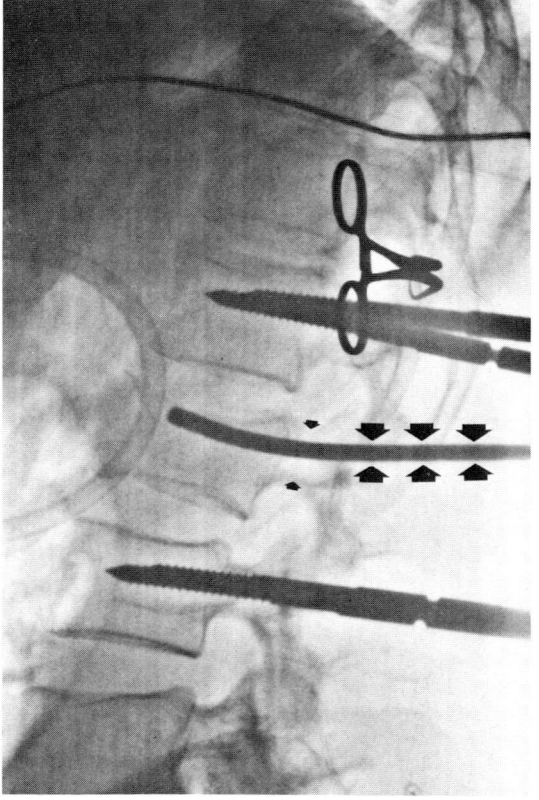

Fig. 33. L2 fracture. Intraoperative radiograph with the punch placed through the pedicle of L2 prior to transpedicular cancellous bone grafting. In L1 and L3 the Schanz screws have already been inserted ready to apply the internal fixator (patient A. W., male, 49 years old).

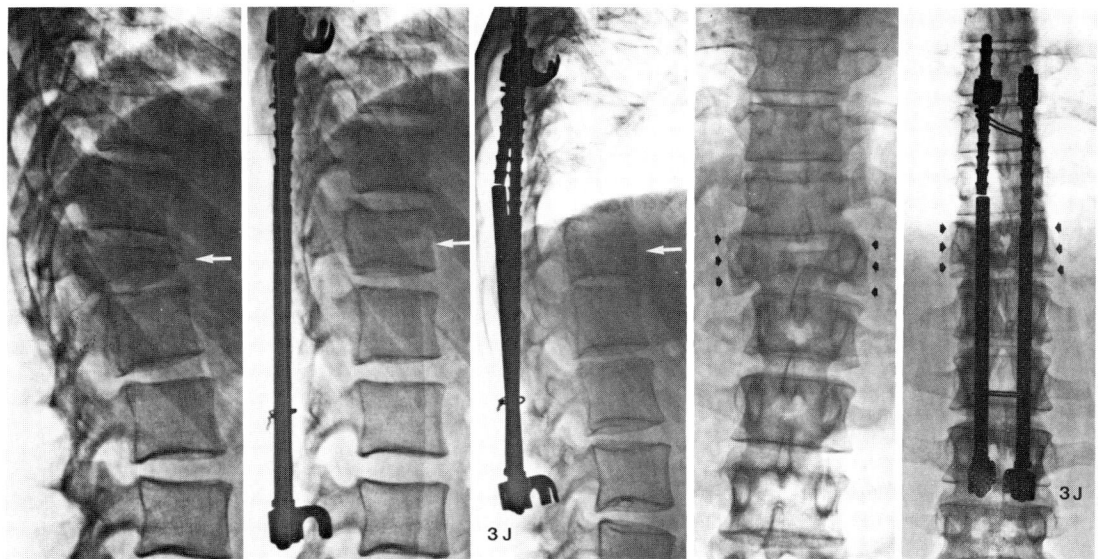

Fig. 34. L1 fracture shown in Figure 8 with fracture healing in a good position. Intraoperatively dorsal fusion from T12–L2. Patient refused implant removal. Three years postoperatively fatigue fracture of one Harrington rod (patient H.A., male, 22 years old).

## 5. Unresolved problems

Most types of instrumentation of vertebral fractures have serious problems in common. These are not due to complications or technical difficulties: complications can never be eliminated completely in medicine, but are not the rule and are avoidable at least in theory. What is meant are rather disadvantages inherent in the various systems due to biomechanical deficiencies which cannot be avoided even when the implants are perfectly applied. This is predominantly the long distance of fixation. The methods in which only a short-range fixation is carried out such as in monosegmental Harrington compression instrumentation can only occasionally be used due to the rarity of suitable fracture types. Anterior bone grafting, use of the Weiss spring or anterior plate fixation all have their own problems. Objections to the use of the external fixator, which can be applied in so many situations biomechanically, are discussed in Section 4. All other systems used more frequently cross four to six motion segments, because they require three or four-point fixation. These include distraction rods, posterior plates, (except

the newest Roy-Camille lumbar spinal plates [167]), Luque instrumentation and long compression instrumentation. The effect of blocking healthy joints which would be inconceivable in the limbs is regarded as functionally insignificant and unavoidable in surgical treatment of the spine, but is this really the case?

We are used to carrying out correction of deformity in spinal fusion over many vertebrae in severe scoliosis without the patient noticing a significant reduction in function in everyday life. However, this experience cannot simply be translated to patients with vertebral fractures, since the fusion in patients with scoliosis does not involve a freely mobile spine, but a spine with slowly increasing loss of function which has occurred over a long period of time, and to which the patient has adapted and developed compensatory mechanisms.

LOUIS [107] compiled the known data on the mobility of the spine and its segments as follows:

Thoracic spine: total flexion – extension 50°
(flexion 30°, extension 20°)
total rotation 70° (2×35°), segments Th1–Th6:

47

6° each, Th6/7: 8°, Th7–Th10: 4° each,
Th10/11: 6°, Th11/12: 4°, Th12/L1: 10°
Total lateral tilting 40° (2×20°).

Lumbar spine: total flexion – extension 83°
(flexion 53°, extension 30°).
segments L1/2: 11°, L2/3: 12°, L3/4: 18°,
L4/5: 24°, L5/S1: 18°
total rotation 16° (2×8°)
total lateral tilting 40° (2×20°)

A loss of four, five or even six segments thus probably gives rise to a significant restriction in mobility, although of course this depends on the level of the instrumentation. A patient without paralysis learns to compensate for this loss, yet it can be irksome, particularly when the lumbar lordosis is abolished, because this leads to alteration in the pattern of gait (WASYLENKO et al. [201]), to hip hyperextension and often to pain, as has been pointed out by HASDAY et al. [73]. However, the situation is very different for the paraplegic, who relies on considerable mobility of the spine particularly in the lumbar region in order to reach a high degree of rehabilitation. There is increasing evidence from paraplegic centers that patients with long fusions of the spine can be mobilized more rapidly [33, 81], but that the final results attained in patients treated conservatively where mobility of the spine is preserved are better, and these patients regain better independence [183, 219]:

- If sitting balance is not very good, a paraplegic cannot reach his foot by raising and pulling the leg up with the arm, but he must bend forwards longitudinally in order to reach his toes with his hands. If flexion of the lumbar spine is impossible, he needs to fold forwards at his hip joints like a pocket knife, and the degree of flexion of the hips may be insufficient to allow this.
- In order to be able to lift objects from the floor whilst sitting in a wheel chair, extensive mobility of the spine is necessary.
- Getting back into the wheelchair after a fall without the help of another person is almost impossible with a stiff lumbar spine or with a corset.
- In order to bring the legs forward in walking exercises using splints, the pelvis must be appropriately tilted using diagonal shortening of the oblique abdominal musculature, which

is more difficult where the lumbar spine is arthrodesed.
- In standing training, the pelvis is pushed forward and the spine is extended in order to balance. It is noticeable that patients with long implants complain about pain doing this, in spite of their loss of sensitivity.
- Where there is ectopic ossification around the hip joint, the ability to sit may depend on mobility of the lumbar spine.

These difficulties are accentuated further if a full-contact corset is necessary to immobilize the entire thoracic and vertebral column postoperatively. A patient without paralysis can compensate by active movement of the lower limbs, but a paraplegic may only be able to undertake the final phases of rehabilitation after removal of the corset, although he can be got out of bed early after operation.

Is the opposite view of E. LUQUE [111] consistent with these observations, however? In fractures of the thoracolumbar junction with complete paraplegia, he aims to carry out very long fusions distally including the sacrum. This is understandable from the social background of his patients in Mexico, which was the reason for developing sublaminar segmental spinal instrumentation. In these cases, it is important to achieve early corset-free sitting without sophisticated rehabilitation and long term followup care.

Theoretically, the problem of immobilization of many motion segments is solved finally after metal removal where only a «short fusion» has been performed at the fracture site. However, this needs more extensive examination, since there are certain quite reasonable theoretical objections. Firstly, HOLM and NACHEMSON [79] showed a loss of water content and a reduction of metabolic processes (i.e. degenerative ageing manifestations) in animal models when uninjured intervertebral discs were immobilized. Secondly, there is no reason why intervertebral joints should show any fundamentally different behavior from peripheral joints. Because of the risk of immobilization damage, limb traumatology attempted to abandon plaster fixation of uninvolved joints in favor of functional treatment, although the immobilization only lasted a few weeks and not 9 to 12 months and there was no postoperative scarring around the joint.

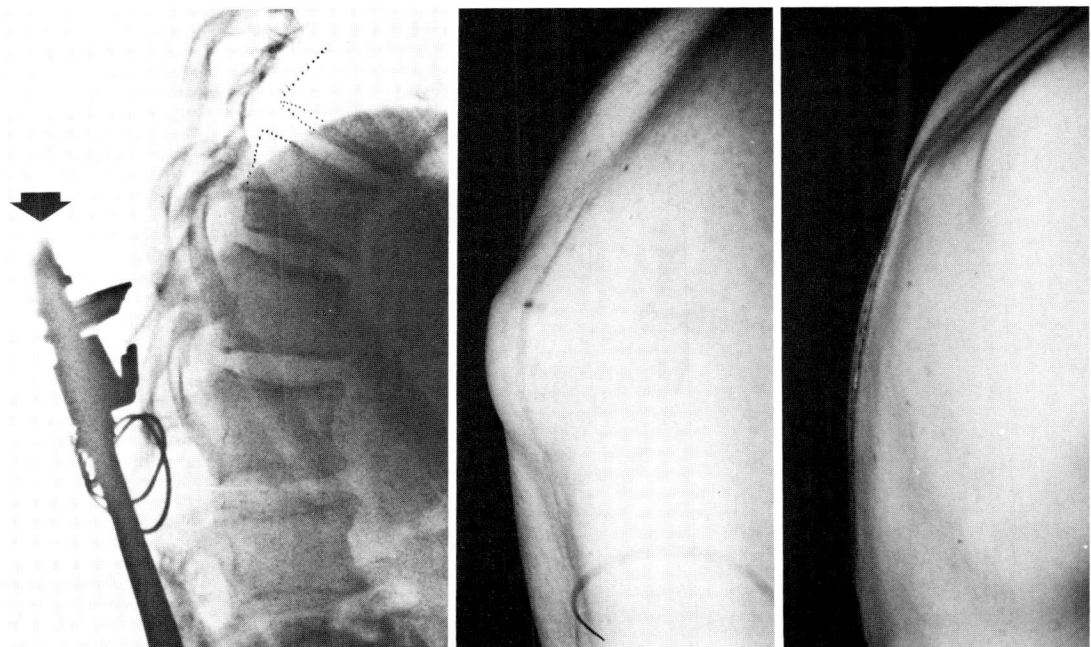

Abb. 35. Example of displaced distraction rod ends with formation of a bursa. On the right, after exchanging the implant for an internal fixator (patient Z.A., male, 22 years old).

Examination of spinal mobility after removal of long rods or plates with functional radiographs at a late stage showed a reduction in mobility between vertebrae compared to normal values. Indeed, not uncommonly one is forced to chisel out the rod from a bony mass stretching the whole length of the rod in order to remove it, even though a short fusion was originally performed. HASDAY et al. [73] also observed reduced mobility of the spine with spontaneous fusion using the «long rod – short fusion» technique. KAHANOVITZ et al. [89, 90] reported similar results in animal experiments as well as clinically.

In implant systems where the vertebrae have a mobile attachment to the longitudinal load carriers, for example in Harrington, Jacobs and Luque rods, the first and second non-instrumented vertebrae above the fixation may move a relatively large distance in anterior flexion. This causes projection of the rod if it protrudes some way proximal to the hooks (Fig. 35), and this may even occur without detachment of the hook. By its movement backwards and forwards in the paraspinal musculature, a large bursa is occasionally formed. With removal of the metal, this disturbing protruberance naturally disappears.

# 6. The «internal fixator» as a new stabilization system

## 6.1 Objectives

A synopsis of the unsolved problems with the advantages and disadvantages of the available fixation systems led to the idea that fundamental improvements were needed in surgical stabilization for fractures of the lower thoracic and lumbar spine. This is particularly true for injuries where there is paraplegia, because the disadvantages of these fixation techniques are especially pronounced during their rehabilitation.

The objectives in developing a fixation system resulting from weaknesses in other systems are as follows:
- The fixation should only include the vertebrae immediately adjacent to the fracture, and the fixation thus should not involve more than two motion segments.
- The system should be versatile, and of use in most different types of fractures.
- The system should provide a method for fracture reduction.

49

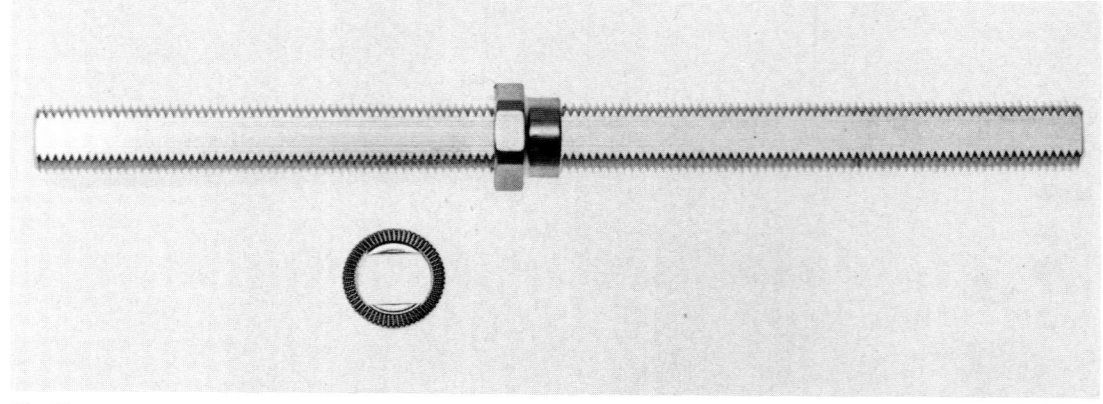

Fig. 36

- The system should be applicable in cases where there has been a prior laminectomy.
- The fixation should require as few special instruments and size graduations as possible.
- The system should be implantable and should not require additional external fixation by full-contact corsets for mobilization.

Besides these, the requirements of Section 2 naturally also apply.

To date, the external fixator most adequately fulfills this catalogue of requirements. MAGERL [120] also planned an implantable device at the start of the development of the external fixator, using transpedicular screws connected to each other, but he then concentrated on external fixation of Schanz screws. He should thus be credited with originating the idea, although the system to be described here was developed independently.

The internal fixator was developed as a new system for stabilization of the spine in collaboration with the instrument factory Mathys[1]. It was first employed clinically on December 23rd 1982. It later became known that KLUGER had already conceived an implant which was in principle the same and which is also being used clinically in the meantime [97].

KRAG et al. [100] and SUEZAWA and JACOB [188] published further descriptions.

[1] R. Mathys, Surgical Instrument Factory, CH–2544 Bettlach, Switzerland.

## 6.2 Technical description

The internal fixator consists of a 10 cm long threaded steel rod with a diameter of 7 mm. The threaded rod is flattened on two sides. This serves first to prevent spontaneous loosening of the nuts, as the collar of the nuts is crimped together at the end of mounting. The collar is sufficiently deformable to allow detachment of the nuts with the wrench for implant removal.

Secondly, the flattening of the rod allows mounting of a washer with an appropriately shaped hole which consequently does not allow rotation. This washer is radially serrated, and interdigitates with an identical serration on the clamp element, thereby preventing rotation of the clamp element. The grooves are placed at 6° intervals. The clamp element carries a clamp on a similarly flattened threaded bolt with similar radial grooves which can rotate freely but can be fixed by a nut.

The clamp is designed in such a way that tightening of the corresponding nut prevents rotation of the clamp and firmly grips the transpedicular screw. An identical assembly is mounted on the other end of the longitudinal rod.

Special 5 mm diameter Schanz screws with a self-cutting thread connect the fixator to the spine. The thread on the screws terminates without a sharp rise of the core diameter to avoid stress rising. The long shafts of the Schanz screws afford excellent lever arms for manual or instrumental fractures reduction. Finally, the dorsally projecting parts of the screws are cut off

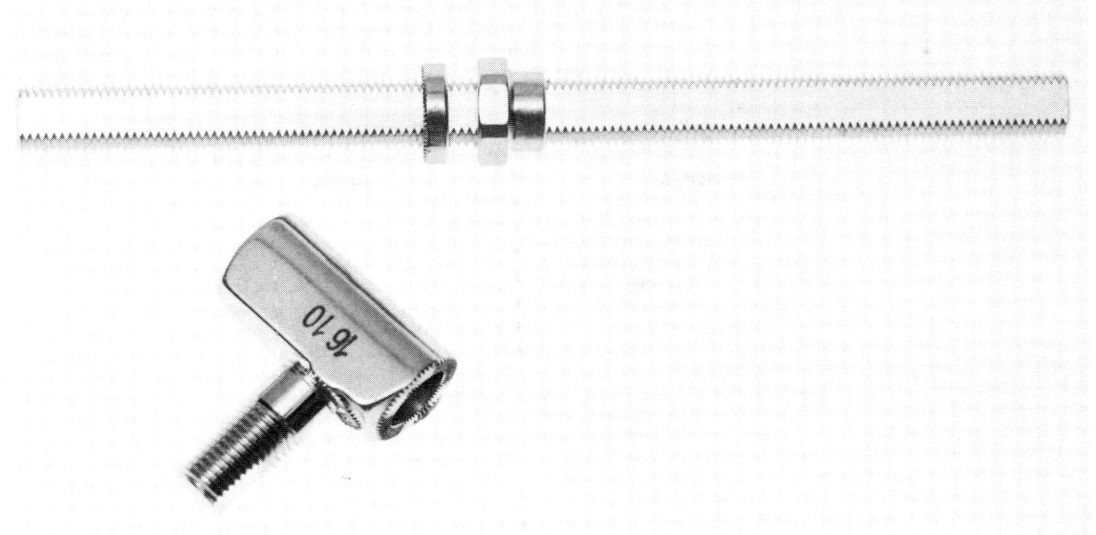

Fig. 37

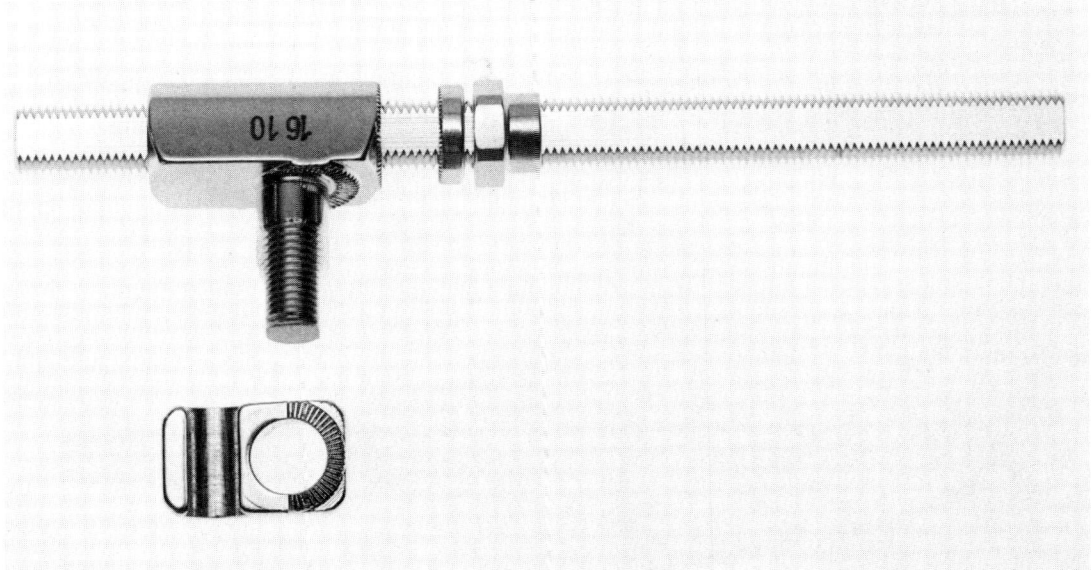

Fig. 38

near to the clamp element with a special bolt cutter.

Use of the large Harrington cutter is not recommended because it is difficult to be positioned, it leaves behind a sharp edge where the screw is cut and causes a severe jerk in the process of cutting. The system of clamp elements and clamps results in free mobility of the internal fixator in three dimensions, which is essential since the direction of the screws is preordained by the anatomy of the pedicles. The Schanz screws cannot be inserted in parallel, for example in the frontal and sagittal planes.

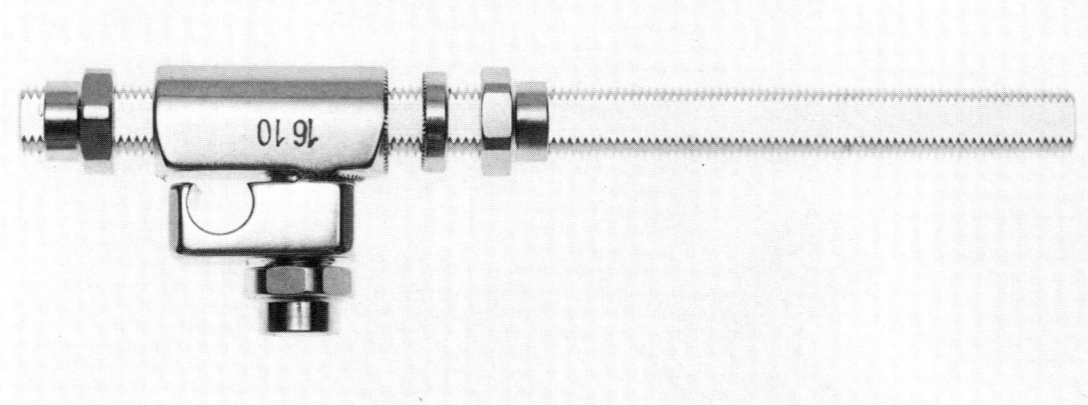

Fig. 39

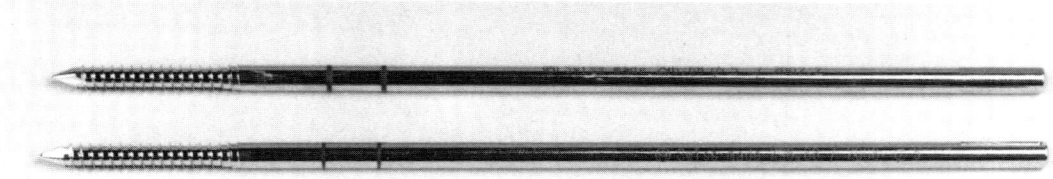

Fig. 40

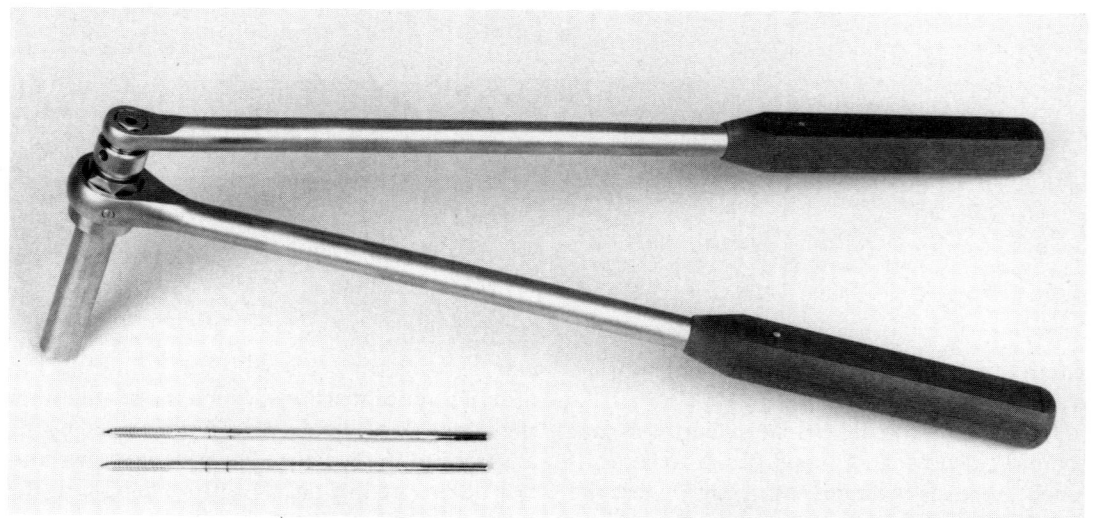

Fig. 41. Bolt cutter for cutting off the ends of the Schanz screws.

52

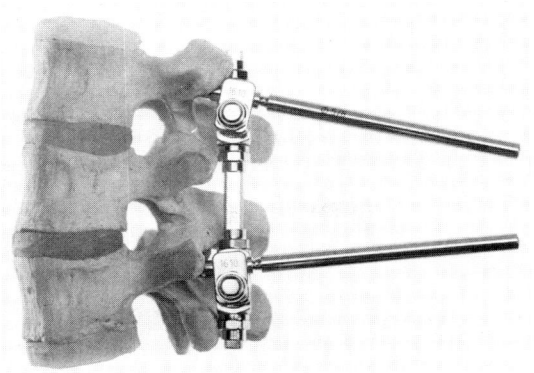

Fig. 42

The standard size of the threaded rods allows for fixation of three vertebrae (Fig. 43). Shorter and longer rods are available.

## 6.3 Biomechanical principles

The internal fixator is the only implantable device in which there is no movement between the longitudinal load carrier and the anchoring device in the vertebrae, once implanted. As it is stable in itself, no further bony support is necessary, apart from the stable positioning of the Schanz screws through the pedicles into the vertebral bodies. Hence the device can be restricted to the vertebrae adjacent to the injured vertebra, and is neither dependent on the anterior longitudinal ligament nor on the posterior wall of the vertebral body nor on the integrity of the posterior column. Using the threaded rod, distraction, compression or neutralization are possible. Unlike the Harrington rod, distraction does not simultaneously lead to a kyphotic force on the terminal vertebrae. Because of the fixed angle between the longitudinal rod and the pedicular screws, parallel distraction or compression are possible. Further, due to the long lever arm of the screws, lordotic correction of the vertebral bodies can be attained by pushing the ends of the Schanz screws together, the clamps not yet being tightened. Conversely, a kyphotic force, for example on a bone graft can be achieved by pressing apart the ends of the screws. By tightening the clamps, compression or tension forces on the vertebral bodies can be fixed within the elasticity of the system. Once

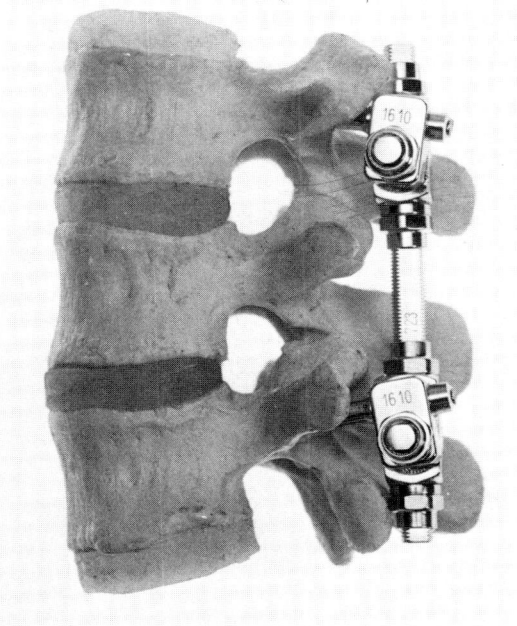

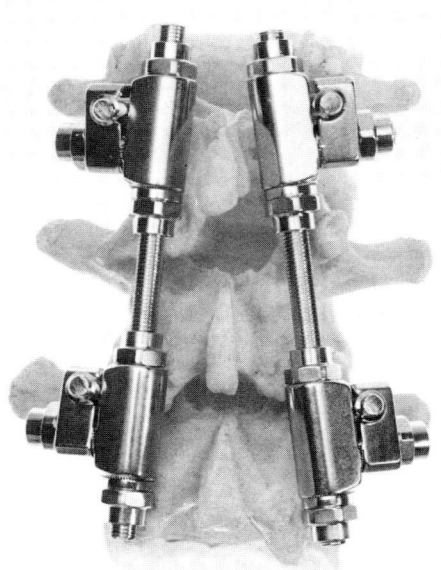

Fig. 43

the tightening nuts have been secured, the instrumented vertebra is safe against flexion-extension forces, axial compression, rotation and anteroposterior shearing forces, limited only by the intrinsic stability of the fixator and the purchase of the screws in the bone. Similar to a bookcase without a back or diagonal struts, it affords little stability against pure lateral movement, in contrast to the external fixator. This is because it is not a closed framework but consists of two separate implants to the right and left of the spinous processes, and the screws remain rotatable in the bone (Fig. 43). Because of the anatomy, such lateral movement is only possible either when the articular processes are broken, when there has been dislocation of the articular processes, or when there is severe comminution of the vertebral body.

Where there is marked instability, the system can be «closed» by a cross-linking device currently being tested, or less effectively by placing diagonal cerclage wires around the Schanz screws. These cross-links then prevent tilting of

the threaded rods from a rectangle to a parallelogram.

However, if the Schanz screws have been inserted convergently towards the midline, a certain stabilization against lateral displacement will have already been achieved without diagonal wiring [97].

## 7. Experimental investigation of the stability of the internal fixator

There are forces and moments acting on the spine *in vivo* which occur with 6 degrees of freedom. The absolute values of these forces and moments *in vivo* are not known. Experimental work to study the stability of spinal specimens so far only took into account single forces or moments in isolation, and was mostly restricted to anterior flexion moments in the literature [4, 83, 84, 94, 101, 141, 153, 186, 214]. The value of these measurements is mainly to test different

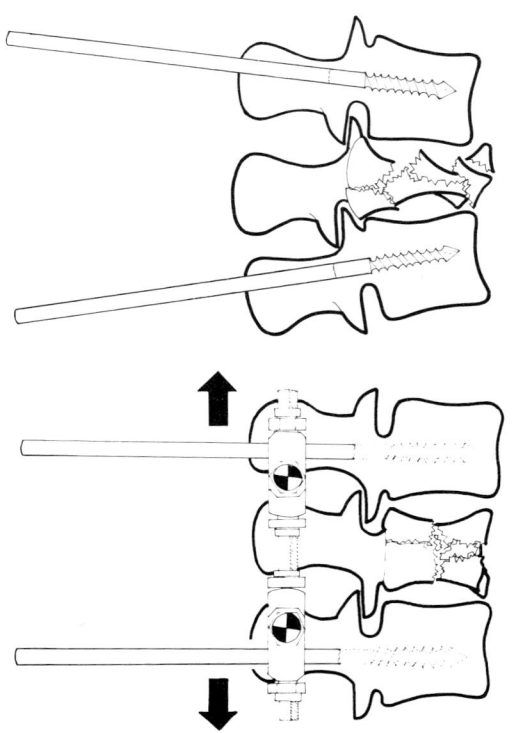
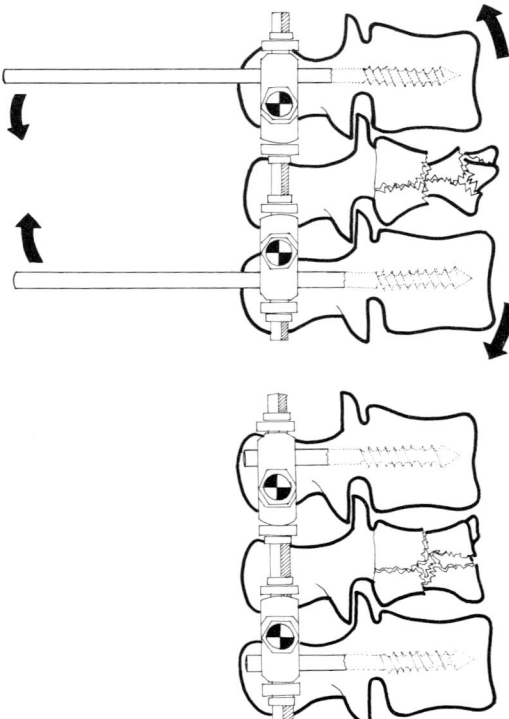

Fig. 44. Principle of action of the internal fixator.

implant techniques using the same system, rather than having any value regarding absolute measurement. Because different investigators work under different experimental conditions, comparisons are rarely possible. For this reason, the same experimental arrangement was used in testing the internal fixator as that used by WÖRSDÖRFER [214] in a series of other implants. In this way, we are able to make comparisons.

## 7.1 Elastic and plastic deformation

In preliminary experimentation, the deformation behavior of the internal fixator was investigated by axial loading of the Schanz screws. The implant was mounted in pairs on two polyethylene blocks separated from each other as shown in Figure 45. The lower block was suspended from the base of the materials testing machine, and the upper block was exposed to continuously rising or falling loads via the spindle drive of the machine. The distance covered was recorded simultaneously and the values plotted on a three-channel plotter. Bending of the entire system in relation to increasing and decreasing loads was measured, as was the deformation remaining at the end of the experiment (if present). To avoid lateral deviation of the polyethylene blocks, the internal fixator was

Table 1

| Flexion moment Nm | distance a with increasing flexion moment mm | distance a with decreasing flexion moment (hysteresis) mm |
|---|---|---|
| .00000 | .00000 | .00000 |
| 1.25000 | .14850 | .33000 |
| 2.50000 | .34650 | .62700 |
| 3.75000 | .54450 | .87450 |
| 5.00000 | .70950 | 1.12200 |
| 6.25000 | .90750 | 1.35300 |
| 7.50000 | 1.07250 | 1.50150 |
| 8.75000 | 1.23750 | 1.65000 |
| 10.00000 | 1.40250 | 1.79850 |
| 11.25000 | 1.56750 | 1.91400 |
| 12.50000 | 1.73250 | 2.06250 |
| 13.75000 | 1.89750 | 2.17800 |
| 15.00000 | 2.06250 | 2.26050 |
| 16.25000 | 2.22750 | 2.37600 |
| 17.50000 | 2.39250 | 2.47500 |
| 18.75000 | 2.55750 | 2.55750 |

secured by diagonal cerclage wires around the Schanz screws as described in section 6.3.

Results: With loading with a flexion moment of up to 18.57 Nm, there was a linear decrease in the distance between the tips of the Schanz screws of 2.56 mm. The hysteresis curve on removal of the load returned to zero, i.e. there was no plastic deformation of the system. This was reproduced identically on three separate runs.

Exactly the same applied with loads up to 25 Nm with a deflection of 3.43 mm and with loads up to 35 Nm with deflection of 4.67 mm. Again, identical results were recorded when the procedure was repeated three times (see appen-

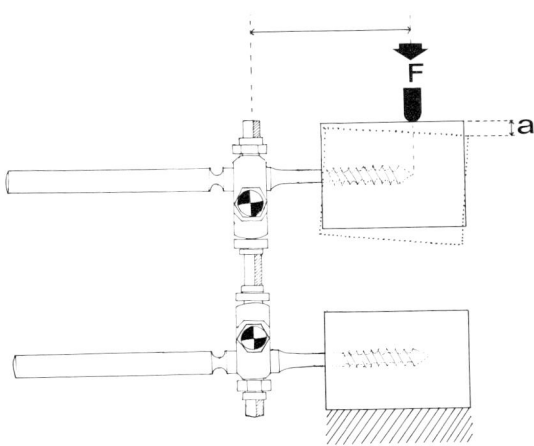

Fig. 45. Test of the deformation of the internal fixator. Mounting on two contact-free polyethylene blocks. The distance between the clamp element and the tips of the Schanz screws, where a force F is applied is 5 cm. Force F and the deflection a are measured, the flexion moment acting on the fixator is calculated.

Table 2

| Flexion moment Nm | distance a with increasing flexion moment mm | distance a with decreasing flexion moment (hysteresis) mm |
|---|---|---|
| .00000 | .00000 | .29700 |
| 2.50000 | .39600 | 1.22100 |
| 5.00000 | .72600 | 1.81500 |
| 7.50000 | 1.07250 | 2.37600 |
| 10.00000 | 1.41900 | 2.93700 |
| 12.50000 | 1.78200 | 3.36600 |
| 15.00000 | 2.11200 | 3.69600 |
| 17.50000 | 2.47500 | 3.96000 |
| 20.00000 | 2.77200 | 4.22400 |
| 22.50000 | 3.06900 | 4.42200 |
| 25.00000 | 3.36600 | 4.75200 |
| 27.50000 | 3.69600 | 4.98300 |
| 30.00000 | 3.99300 | 5.24700 |
| 32.50000 | 4.29000 | 5.47800 |
| 35.00000 | 4.58700 | 5.70900 |
| 37.50000 | 4.85100 | 5.94000 |
| 40.00000 | 5.14800 | 6.17100 |
| 42.50000 | 5.41200 | 6.40200 |
| 45.00000 | 5.70900 | 6.63300 |
| 47.50000 | 6.00600 | 6.89700 |
| 50.00000 | 6.27000 | 7.09500 |
| 52.50000 | 6.56700 | 7.32600 |
| 55.00000 | 6.83100 | 7.55700 |
| 57.50000 | 7.12800 | 7.75500 |
| 60.00000 | 7.42500 | 7.95300 |
| 62.50000 | 7.72200 | 8.18400 |
| 65.00000 | 8.01900 | 8.38200 |
| 67.50000 | 8.31600 | 8.51400 |
| 70.00000 | 8.61300 | 8.61300 |

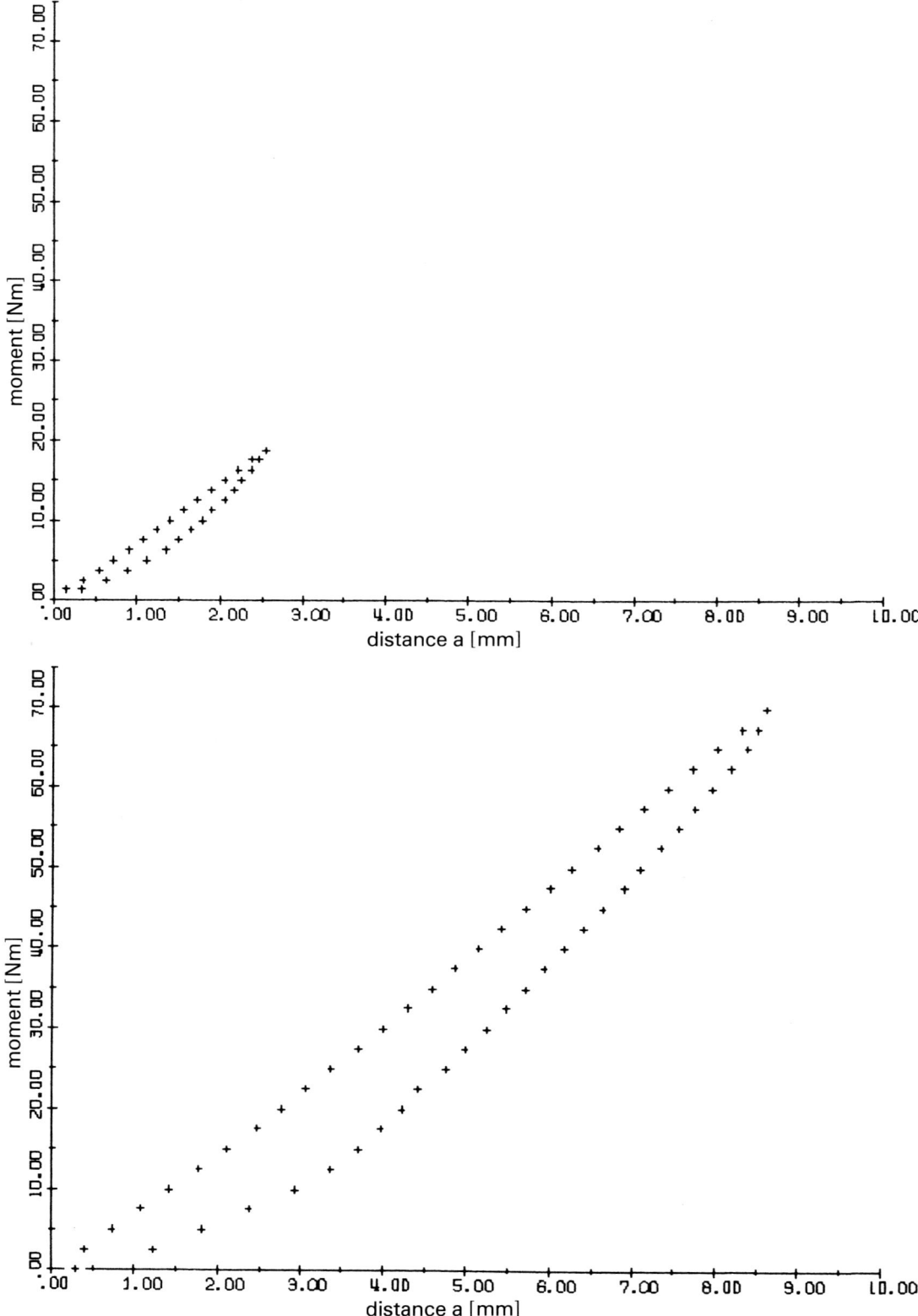

56

Fig. 46. Deflection (a) in relation to the flexion moment occuring in the experimental setting shown in Figure 45. The upper straight line shows the values as the flexion moment is increased, the lower curve shows the return to zero as the flexion moment is decreased (hysteresis).

dix Section 11). The hysteresis curve did not return to zero with a load fo 42.5 Nm and a deflection of 5.46 mm. Here, a plastic deformation of 0.16 mm was registered. Thus the elastic range of the system was exceeded with this load (see appendix Section 11).

With a load of 70 Nm, a deflection of 8.61 mm was recorded, and the plastic deformation was 0.3 mm. Loosening of the clamps did not occur.

To summarize, the experiments show that the implant undergoes linear deflection of around 5 mm in axial loading of the Schanz screw tips to around 40 Nm, with an elastic recoil to the initial unloaded position. In further loading of 40–70 Nm, there is plastic deformation which led to persistent deflection of up to 0.3 mm.

### 7.2 Flexion stability in the fracture model

The stability of the internal fixator in flexion was tested on spinal specimens which had been fractured postmortem. Angular deformity in the region of the fracture was compared to a defined pure flexion moment, and this was chosen as the yardstick for stability as described by WÖRS-DÖRFER [214].

Seven spinal specimens of T11/L5 were harvested from autopsies in unselected patients without known tumor metastases, all being elderly individuals with corresponding porosis. The specimens were freed of muscle and frozen at –20 °C without any other fixative. For the experiments, they were thawed to room temperature and reinforced with multiple screws at either end for better attachment, the heads of the screws projecting into a mould. The two cranial and two caudal terminal vertebrae were cast into self-hardening plastic (methylmethacrylate, Beracryl®). The specimens were then placed in the materials testing machine and loaded with a flexion moment whilst intact. A fracture of L2 or L3

was then performed, and it was decided to test the fixator with a maximal lesion so that a combined anterior and posterior injury was made. A wedge resection was taken from the vertebral body including the posterior vertebral wall, leaving behind the anterior longitudinal ligament.

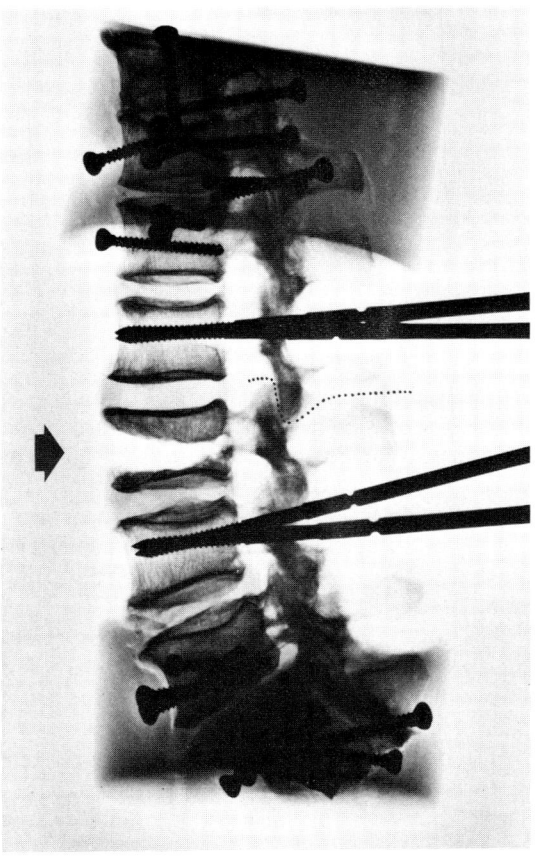

Fig. 48. Spinal specimen where a fracture gap has been created in L3 (arrow) with a dorsal lesion. The ends of the specimen are cast in bone cement after placing reinforcing screws which project from the vertebrae at the end of the specimen. The Schanz screws have been inserted into L2 and L4 but are not yet connected to the internal fixator.

Fig. 47. Deflection (a) in relation to the flexion moment in the experimental setting shown in Figure 45. The upper straight line shows the values as the flexion moment is increased, the lower curve shows the return as the flexion moment is decreased (hysteresis). The line does not return to zero, revealing persistent deformation of 0.3 mm.

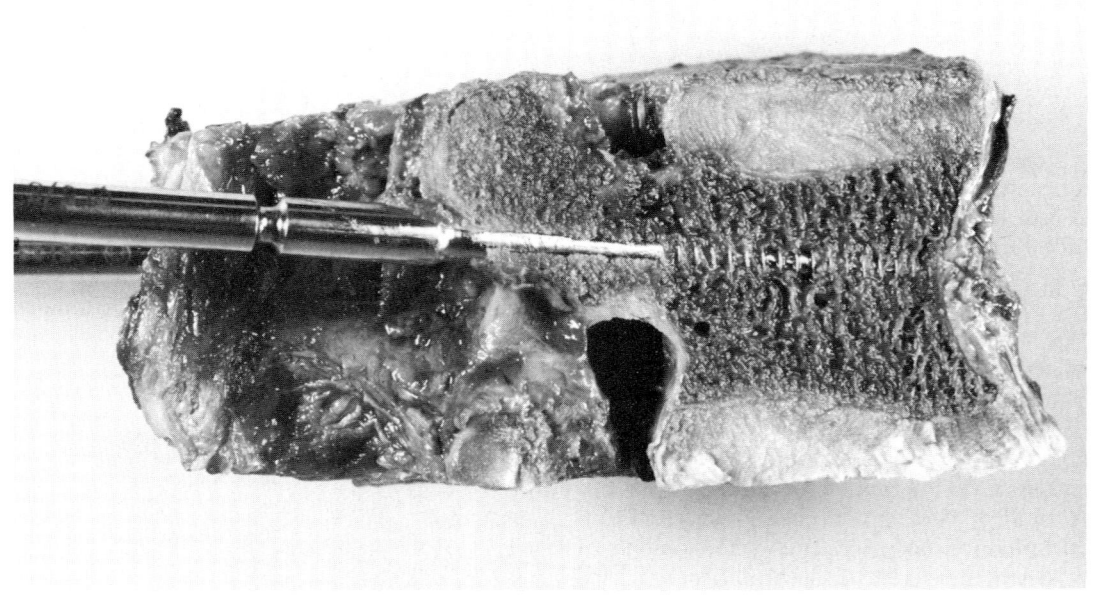

Fig. 49. Firm anchorage of the Schanz screws in specimen S2 after stressing it with a flexion moment of 47.5 Nm.

Dorsally, the interspinous ligaments, the capsule of the specimen vertebral joint, the ligamentum flavum and the posterior longitudinal ligament were divided. Once this was performed, very slight flexion stress caused complete separation of the vertebrae. The fixator was then mounted on the specimen without diagonal wire suspension.

The results of individual experimental measurements on the seven spinal specimens are shown in the form of tables and graphs in the appendix in Section 11.

Specimen S2 was loaded to 47.5 Nm and afterwards sawn apart along the Schanz screws. These showed a firm fit (Fig. 49). There was a residual plastic angular deformity of 0.3°.

In specimen S4, there was a slow yield of the bone around the Schanz screws at about 12 Nm. There had been some alteration of the bone by autolysis. Thus there was increased angulation without detachment of the screws. Figure 50 shows the cavitation in the bone in the section around the Schanz screw and the tilting movement after 20 Nm of flexion stress which had caused this. Figures 51 to 53 show superimposi-

tion of the curves of the specimens S1–7 and a specimen from Section 7.3.

### 7.3 Flexion stability of an *in vivo* instrumentation

One patient, a 43-year-old male, died of a pulmonary embolism 17 days after implantation of the internal fixator, whilst mobilizing. The patient had a four week old, very severe, fracture dislocation with a comminuted fracture of T12, with destruction of the anterior and posterior columns, and an irreversible spinal cord lesion (Fig. 54). Thus restoration of the vertebral height by distraction was dispensed with for the sake of rapid consolidation. At autopsy, the spinal region with the internal fixator in position was removed and frozen at –20 °C. After thawing at room temperature, the spine was subjected to a flexion stress up to the extreme of 47 Nm, using the material testing machine. This was done as described above without any manipulation of the internal fixator. There was elastic deformation of the fixator with return to zero of the hysteresis curve. Afterwards, the clamps of the

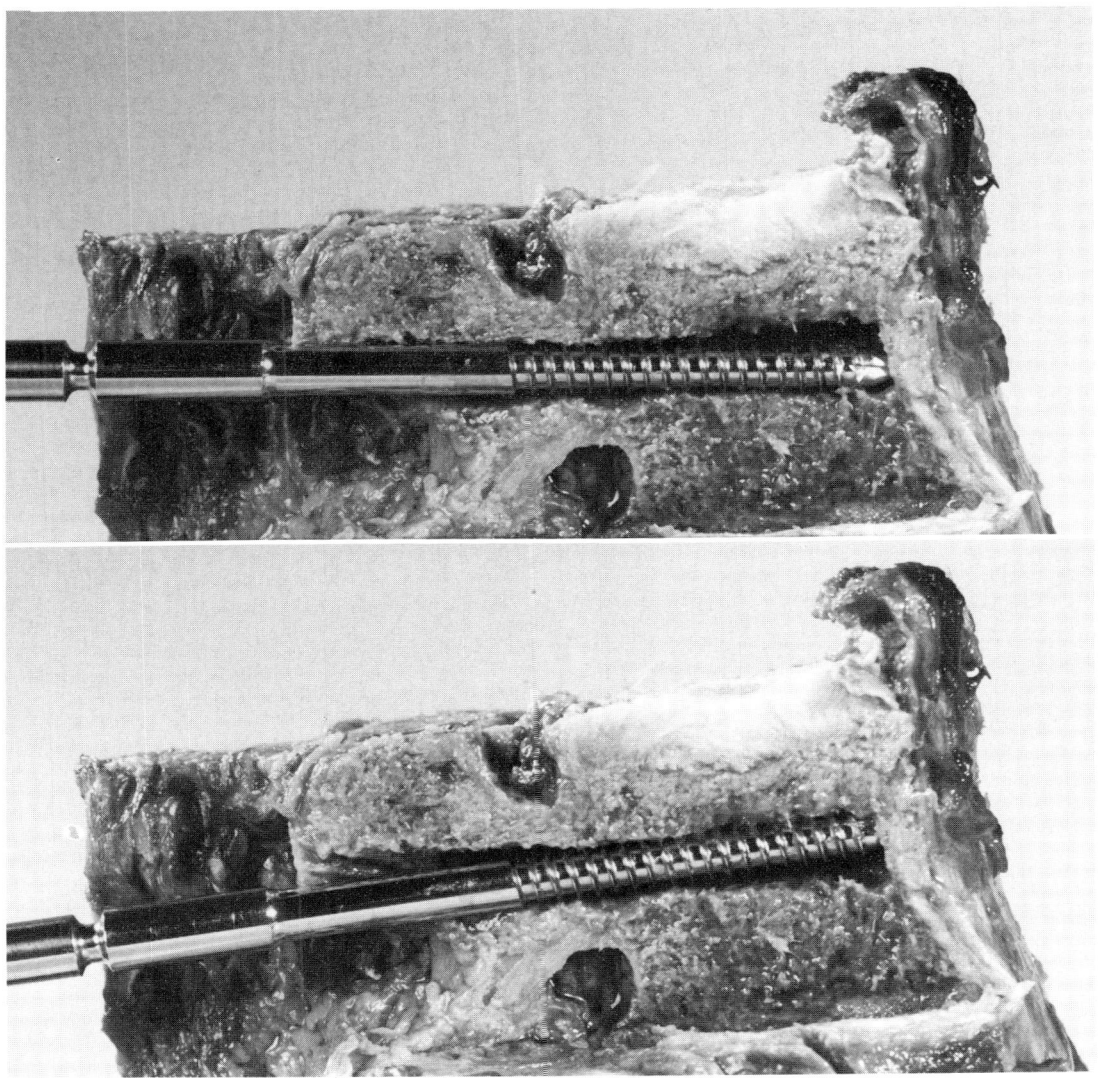

Fig. 50. Specimen S4. After stressing with a flexion moment of 20 Nm, the Schanz screws have moved and tilted within the cancellous bone: the osteoporotic bone of this 83 year old female patient has yielded.

fixator were detached and the longitudinal threaded rods removed. Flexion stress was reapplied without the fixator, and the spine broke in two at about 9 Nm (Fig. 56). The vertebral body was then cut through horizontally, and the position of the Schanz screws in the bone was checked. The emplacement in the pedicles was correct, and the screws were perfectly stable even after loading of 47 Nm (Fig. 55).

The following results are worthy of note in this experimental test of a real spinal injury with anterior and posterior lesions stabilized by an internal fixator:
– With a flexion stress of 10 Nm, an angular deformation of 0.9° was measured, at 15 Nm, 1.1°, at 20 Nm, 1.4°, and at 47 Nm, only 2.4°.
– After a flexion stress of 47 Nm, the system returned to the initial position on unloading without any plastic deformation.

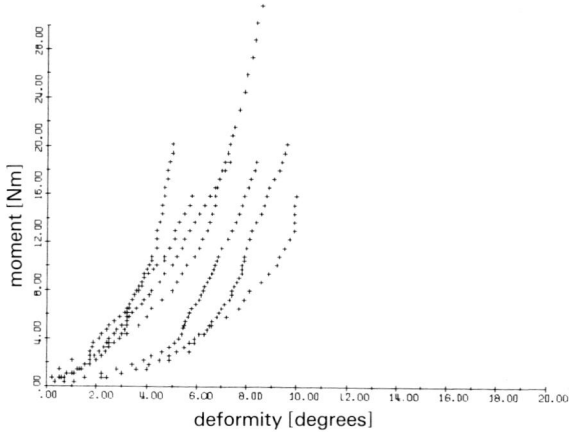

Fig. 51. Superimposition of the curves of intact spines. The figure represents the angular deformation in degrees between adjacent vertebrae prior to injury, in relation to the flexion moment in Nm.

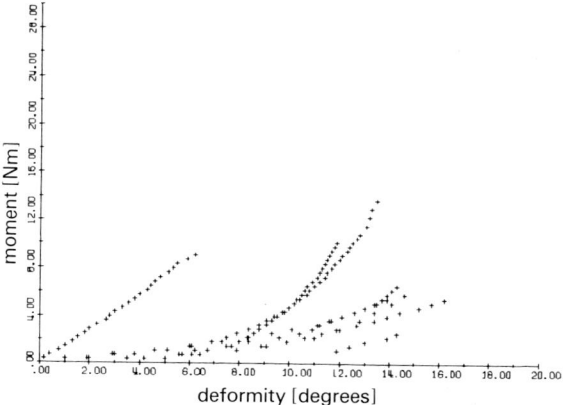

Fig. 52. Superimposition of the curves after combined anterior and posterior lesions have been created.

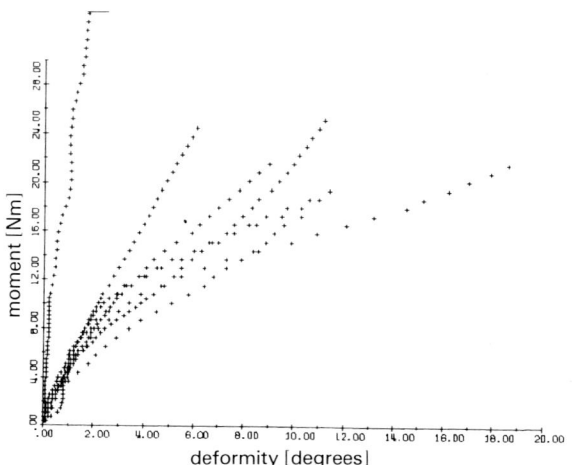

Fig. 53. Superimposition of the curves after mounting the internal fixator.

60

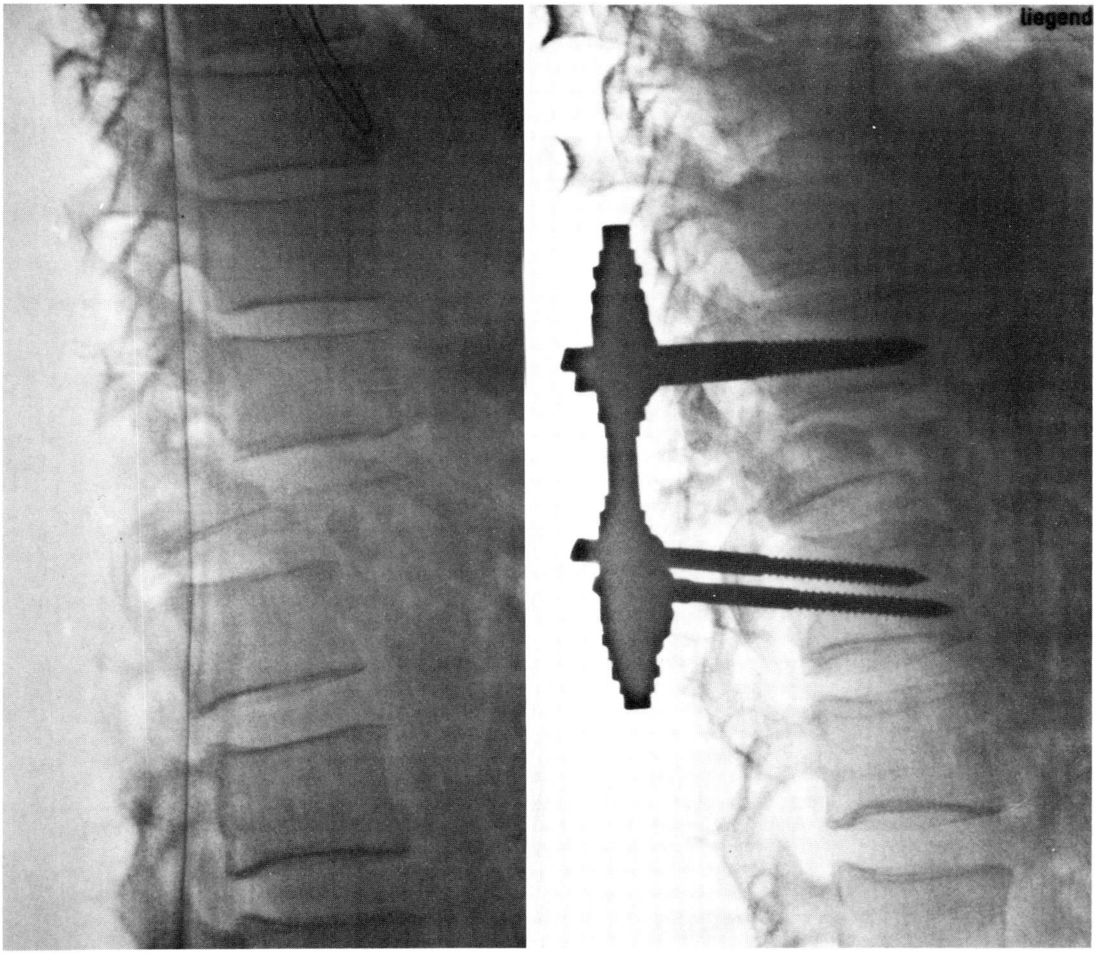

Fig. 54. M.A. (43 year old male). Instrumented four weeks after injury.

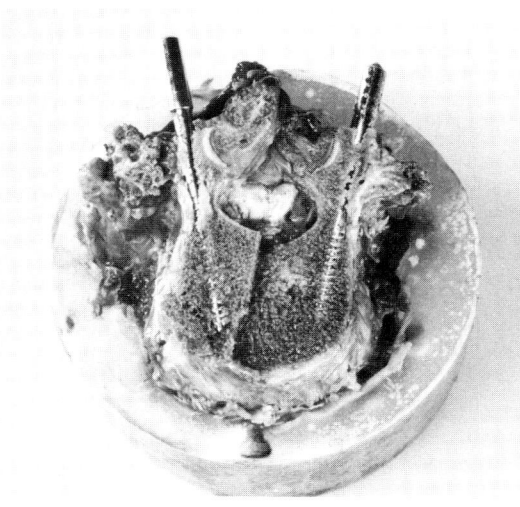

– After this flexion stress, the purchase of the Schanz screws was firm. In other words the bone screw interface and the fixator had only been strained in the elastic range.

– The flexion stress of 47 Nm is several times the flexion moment expected in vivo, according to SCHLÄPFER and WÖRSDÖRFER [172]. For comparison of other experimental lesions of WÖRSDÖRFER [214] and JACOBS et al. [83], the Harrington distraction system dislocated at 6–10 Nm, and the locking hook spinal rod system at 19–35 Nm of flexion stress.

Fig. 55. Spinal specimen of the patient from Figure 54, who died of pulmonary embolism 17 days postoperatively. The specimen has been sawn through horizontally along the screws following testing.

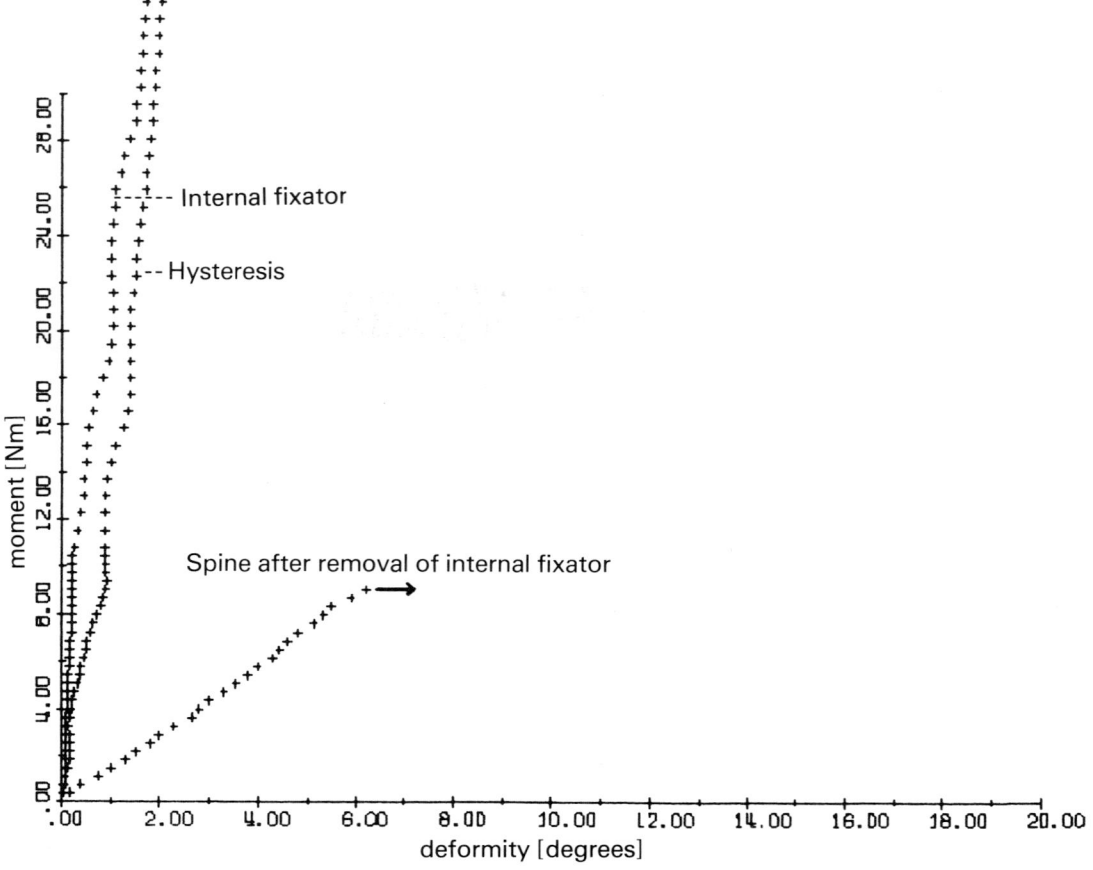

Fig. 56. Specimen of the case shown in Figures 54 and 55. The patient had a severe comminuted fracture with dislocation fixed with the internal fixator. Angular deformation in degrees between the two vertebral bodies adjacent to the fracture in relation to the flexion moment applied in Nm. The right of the two curves of the internal fixator shows hysteresis values returning to zero as the flexion stress is decreased. The arrow designates disruption of the preparation in subsequent testing once the fixator had been removed.

## 7.4 Discussion

Summarizing the experiments above, the following conclusions can be drawn:

– The clamps are able to withstand the flexion moments which probably occur in vivo. The clamps did not fail either using the fixator with the plastic cubes with a flexion moment of 70 Nm with plastic deformation (7.1) nor in the experimental studies using spinal specimens (Sections 7.2.2 and 7.3). The experimental evidence suggests that the connection between the screws and the rods is sufficiently stable, and yet allows movement in three dimensions before nut tightening.

– The connection between the screws and the bone is the limiting factor in stability. However, a screw passing through the pedicle into the vertebral body has an extremely firm hold. Clinical experience has shown that when stresses are too high, the screws break rather than displace, and the vertebra does not fracture. MAGERL saw no loosening of the screws in 49 clinical cases of external fixator [119]. However, the greater elasticity of his system reduces peak stresses on the bone screw interface [214] in comparison to the internal fixator. In the experiments described above using osteoporotic spinal specimens with an average age of 78 years, in only two cases did the

Table 3. Spinal specimen of the patient of Figure 54 and 55 with *in-vivo* internal fixator instrumentation.

| Flexion moment Nm | Angular deformation with increasing flexion moment degrees | Angular deformation with decreasing flexion moment (hysteresis) degrees |
|---|---|---|
| .36000 | .02000 | .00000 |
| .72000 | .05000 | .00000 |
| 1.08000 | .05000 | .05000 |
| 1.44000 | .07000 | .10000 |
| 1.80000 | .07000 | .15000 |
| 2.16000 | .05000 | .17000 |
| 2.52000 | .07000 | .17000 |
| 2.88000 | .07000 | .15000 |
| 3.24000 | .07000 | .10000 |
| 3.60000 | .07000 | .15000 |
| 3.96000 | .10000 | .18000 |
| 4.32000 | .10000 | .20000 |
| 4.68000 | .10000 | .25000 |
| 5.04000 | .10000 | .30000 |
| 5.40000 | .12000 | .35000 |
| 5.76000 | .15000 | .40000 |
| 6.12000 | .15000 | .45000 |
| 6.48000 | .17000 | .50000 |
| 6.84000 | .17000 | .50000 |
| 7.20000 | .20000 | .60000 |
| 7.56000 | .20000 | .65000 |
| 7.92000 | .20000 | .72000 |
| 8.28000 | .20000 | .80000 |
| 8.64000 | .20000 | .85000 |
| 9.00000 | .20000 | .90000 |
| 9.36000 | .20000 | .92000 |
| 9.72000 | .20000 | .90000 |
| 10.08000 | .20000 | .90000 |
| 10.44000 | .20000 | .88000 |
| 10.80000 | .25000 | .88000 |
| 11.52000 | .31000 | .88000 |
| 12.24000 | .40000 | .88000 |
| 12.96000 | .45000 | .90000 |
| 13.68000 | .45000 | .92000 |
| 14.40000 | .50000 | 1.00000 |
| 15.12000 | .50000 | 1.10000 |
| 15.84000 | .55000 | 1.25000 |
| 16.56000 | .65000 | 1.35000 |
| 17.28000 | .70000 | 1.40000 |
| 18.00000 | .85000 | 1.40000 |
| 18.71999 | .95000 | 1.40000 |
| 19.43999 | 1.00000 | 1.40000 |
| 20.15999 | 1.05000 | 1.40000 |
| 20.87999 | 1.05000 | 1.40000 |
| 21.59999 | 1.05000 | 1.45000 |
| 22.31999 | 1.00000 | 1.50000 |
| 23.03999 | 1.00000 | 1.50000 |
| 23.75999 | 1.00000 | 1.55000 |
| 24.48000 | 1.05000 | 1.60000 |
| 25.20000 | 1.10000 | 1.65000 |
| 25.92000 | 1.10000 | 1.70000 |
| 26.64000 | 1.20000 | 1.72000 |
| 27.36000 | 1.27000 | 1.77000 |
| 28.07999 | 1.38000 | 1.80000 |
| 28.79999 | 1.50000 | 1.85000 |
| 29.51999 | 1.50000 | 1.85000 |
| 30.23999 | 1.60000 | 1.90000 |
| 30.95999 | 1.60000 | 1.92000 |
| 31.67999 | 1.63000 | 1.95000 |
| 32.39999 | 1.67000 | 1.96000 |
| 33.12000 | 1.68000 | 2.00000 |
| 33.84000 | 1.70000 | 2.03000 |
| 34.56000 | 1.72000 | 2.07000 |
| 35.28000 | 1.75000 | 2.10000 |
| 36.00000 | 1.80000 | 2.11000 |
| 36.72000 | 1.82000 | 2.14000 |
| 37.43999 | 1.87000 | 2.17000 |
| 38.15999 | 1.90000 | 2.20000 |
| 38.87999 | 1.90000 | 2.22000 |
| 39.59999 | 1.95000 | 2.24000 |
| 40.31999 | 2.00000 | 2.26000 |
| 41.03999 | 2.03000 | 2.29000 |
| 41.75999 | 2.07000 | 2.29000 |
| 42.48000 | 2.12000 | 2.30000 |
| 43.20000 | 2.17000 | 2.31000 |
| 43.92000 | 2.25000 | 2.31000 |
| 44.64000 | 2.27000 | 2.40000 |
| 45.36000 | 2.30000 | 2.40000 |
| 46.08000 | 2.30000 | 2.40000 |
| 46.79999 | 2.35000 | 2.40000 |
| 47.51999 | 2.38000 | 2.40000 |
| 47.87999 | 2.40000 | 2.40000 |

Table 4. Same specimen without internal fixator. Testing of the flexion load-carrying capacity of the fracture. At 9.3 Nm, there is complete disruption of the specimen.

| Flexion moment Nm | Angular deformation after removal of the internal fixator degrees |
|---|---|
| .36000 | .15000 |
| .72000 | .40000 |
| 1.08000 | .75000 |
| 1.44000 | 1.00000 |
| 1.80000 | 1.30000 |
| 2.16000 | 1.50000 |
| 2.52000 | 1.80000 |
| 2.88000 | 2.00000 |
| 3.24000 | 2.30000 |
| 3.60000 | 2.65000 |
| 3.96000 | 2.80000 |
| 4.32000 | 3.00000 |
| 4.68000 | 3.30000 |
| 5.04000 | 3.55000 |
| 5.40000 | 3.80000 |
| 5.76000 | 4.00000 |
| 6.12000 | 4.30000 |
| 6.48000 | 4.45000 |
| 6.84000 | 4.60000 |
| 7.20000 | 4.80000 |
| 7.56000 | 5.15000 |
| 7.92000 | 5.35000 |
| 8.28000 | 5.50000 |
| 8.64000 | 5.90000 |
| 9.00000 | 6.20000 |

**9.36:** complete disruption of the specimen

Schanz screws cut into the cancellous bone of the vertebrae at 12 Nm of flexion stress. In the other specimens, the screw fixation on the bone was still firm even after stresses of 20 and in some cases 40 Nm, whereas using the same experimental model Harrington rods dislocated at 10 Nm (WÖRSDÖRFER [214].

- If the forces applied exceed the anchoring stability of these Schanz screws, they gradually sink into the cancellous bone (S3 and 4). This allows an increase of angulation of the vertebrae without complete loss of stability, as is the case in abrupt dislocational cutting out of Harrington hooks.
- The elastic range of the system is present until approximately 40 Nm of flexion moment.
- The Schanz screws described have a larger diameter (5 mm) compared to screws used with plates, and in the critical region in the pedicle the screws are free of a thread, avoiding undue weakening in this area. The danger of a fracture occurring is thus reduced, although over a longer period of time fracturing may occur.

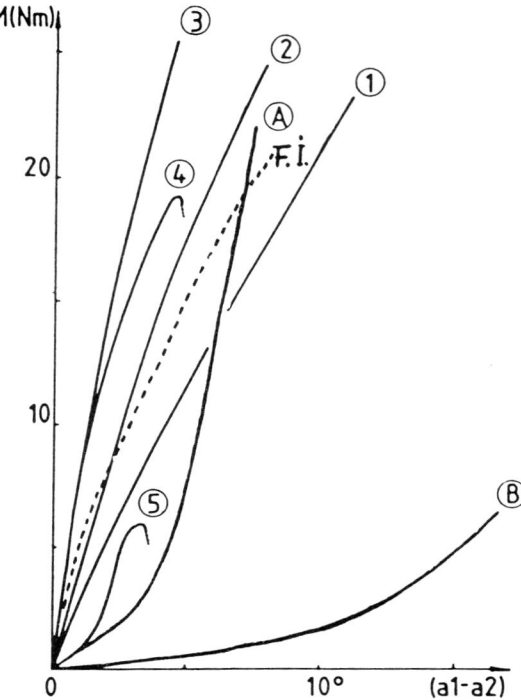

Fig. 57. WÖRSDÖRFER [214]: comparative deformation loading diagrams, A) intact spine, B) combined anterior and posterior instability. 1) external fixator without prestressing, 2) external fixator with prestressing and screw fixation of the intervertebral joints. 3) plate osteosynthesis described by Roy-Camille. 4) locking hook spinal rod distraction system. 5) Harrington distraction system. Dashed curve: Internal fixator.

– In all specimens, the initial angular deformation was less with the internal fixator than in the uninjured spine. With a flexion moment of 14 Nm and higher the angular deformation of the instrumented fracture model exceeded the uninjured spine, except in one case where this already occurred at 11.5 Nm.
– Combining the specimens S1–7 and the specimen in Section 7.3, the average angular deformation at 5 Nm flexion moment is 1°, at 10 Nm 2.9°, at 15 Nm 6.1° and at 20 Nm 6.6°. Thus where the internal fixator is used without screw fixation of the intervertebral joint, the curve of the internal fixator lies between the curves of the external fixator with and without pre-stressing (WÖRSDÖRFER [214]).

Using caution, the following conclusions can be drawn from the available data: the internal fixator displays *at least* the same stability against flexion stresses as the Harrington distraction system and its modifications. The design safeguards against rotation. In view of the advantage of the short fixation distance, the clinical application is hence justified.

More recently, WÖRSDÖRFER [216] and KORT-MANN [98] investigated stability in torsion stress. They have demonstrated that only the external fixator, internal fixator and dorsal plate fixation have adequate rotational stability, and that distraction rods or segmental sublaminar wiring do not protect against rotation.

## 8. Application of the internal fixator in the treatment of vertebral fractures

### 8.1 Surgical technique

The patient should be positioned prone on a Wilson Frame adding Dunlop cushions for prevention of pressure sores in the case of paraplegia. A midline incision is made over five spinous processes. The paraspinal muscles are dissected by subperiosteal dissection as far laterally as the intervertebral joints. Using a shorter incision, wound spreaders or levers may cause pressure necrosis on the soft tissues for adequate lateral dissection. The point of screw entry is identified on the vertebrae adjacent to the fractured vertebra as specified by LOUIS [107], ROY-CAMILLE et al. [163, 164, 165, 166] and SAILLANT [170]. The cranial facet joint and the transverse process are the points of reference. The entry point is placed somewhat further lateral than suggested by ROY-CAMILLE, because the course of the screw is not perpendicular as described by him, but convergent towards the midline.

The precise entry point for the screw is shown in Figure 58a. The entry point in the thoracic spine is just below the intervertebral joint, 3 mm lateral to the center of the joint. The transverse process at this point is beginning to rise posteriorly. It is resected with a rongeur, so that it does not obstruct the clamp element. The point of entry in the lumbar spine is situated on a line passing through the middle of the transverse process

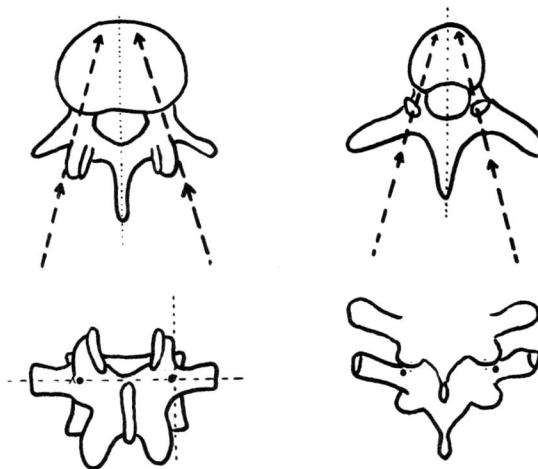

Fig. 58a. Points of entry for the Schanz screws of the internal fixator, on the left for the lumbar spine, on the right for the thoracic spine.

at the lateral edge of the cranial articular process of the vertebra. Even in the lumbar spine, it is often helpful to remove the lower part of the cranial articular process and create a flat area at the entry point. In the sacrum, the entry point is between the L5–S1 joint space and the first sacral foramen, the same point laterally as in the lower lumbar region.

Once the entry points have been determined, a 2 mm Kirschner wire is drilled 10°–15° convergent towards the midline, to a depth of 3 cm and parallel with the end plates. During insertion, one must constantly feel bony contact. Positioning of the wire is checked with the image intensifier. In the lateral projection the level of entry and the direction of the wire in relation to the end plates can be determined. In the AP projection, the tips of the Kirschners wires should converge towards the midline. If the operating table is tilted until the Kirschner wire is vertical in space, and is seen on the image intensifier as a point in its vertical projection, its fit in the pedicle can be determined as the pedicle will be seen as an oval on the X-ray screen [69]. Figure 58b shows a screw hole in this projection, with the screw hole visible in the pedicle a few days after removal of the metal.

When the Kirschner wires are correctly sited, they are replaced one after another by the Schanz

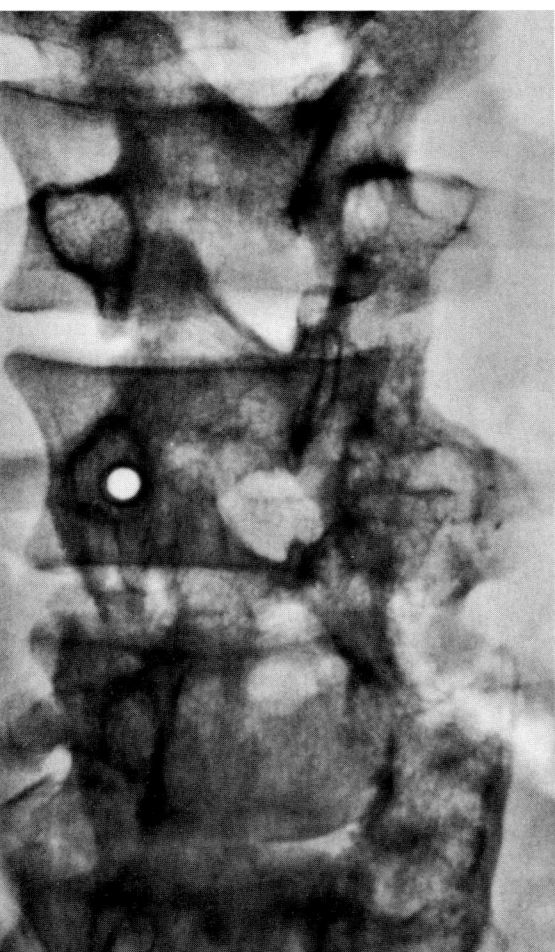

Fig. 58b. A radiograph showing the former course of the Schanz screw through the pedicle of the vertebral body, once the screw has been removed. The radiograph is taken by adjustment of the image intensifier to lie parallel with the course of the screw. The position of the trial Kirschner wire can also be checked in the same way once it has been introduced (patient P. D., male, 19 years old).

screws of the fixator. The first K wire is removed with the power drill and the entry point is opened to a depth of 0,5–1 cm with a 3.5 mm drill bit. It is not drilled deeper and no thread is cut. The self-cutting Schanz screw is then effortlessly screwed in by hand in the same direction as the Kirschner wire before. It goes without saying that a power drill should never be used to do this. The screw can be screwed into a depth of 4 cm in the adult patient except in the sacrum. This can be estimated by the 5 cm mark on the Schanz screws. The remaining screws are placed in the same way.

The screws can be screwed in deeper, but only using the image intensifier. The anterior cortical wall of the vertebral body is thin and gives little resistance so that the surgeon cannot feel the screw perforating the wall. The tip of the screw should be near to or at most in the subcortical bone, but should never pass through the anterior vertebral wall due to the danger of vascular injury. Using the image intensifier, one must be aware of the circular shape of the vertebral body. If a Schanz screw is only slightly convergent, the tip of the screw can easily perforate laterally the vertebral cortex before it appears to reach the anterior wall on the image intensifier. Figure 59 shows correct positioning of the screws.

Our experience would suggest that the screws can be placed to a depth of 4.5 to 5 cm in the thoracic spine below T 8, and 5 to 5.5 cm in the lumbar spine.

The sacrum is different because S 1 is much less wide in the AP plane. Here, particular care must be taken to ensure convergence of the screws, and the maximum depth of penetration is 3 to 3.5 cm.

After emplacement of the four Schanz screws, partial reduction of the fracture can be achieved manually by using the long projecting ends of the screws. In very severe dislocations with massive shortening and lateral displacement, temporary use may be made of an outrigger with hooks placed farther away, or a distraction rod which

is removed afterwards may occasionally be helpful. A pelvic repositioning pliers may also be of assistance.

Next, the threaded rod of the internal fixator with the clamps is placed on the Schanz screws bilaterally, so that the rod comes to rest medially to the screws in the groove between the spinous processes and the vertebral arch. Then reduction of the fracture is performed using the internal fixator. This must always begin with correction of the kyphosis, and vertebral height can only subsequently be restored by distraction. The technique depends on the type of fracture:

*Compression fractures with the posterior wall of the vertebral body intact:* To correct the kyphosis, the dorsal ends of the screws are pressed together until the desired angle of correction has been attained. To do this, the clamp elements must be able to slide freely on the threaded rods, and the distraction nuts must lie in the middle of the rods far away from the clamp elements as shown in Figure 60 No. 5. The center of rotation for the lordosing maneuver is then lying at the posterior edge of the instrumented vertebral body. When the kyphosis has been eliminated, the lateral nuts are tightened on the clamp elements (no. 4 in Fig. 60) and this fixes the angle between the longitudinal rod and the Schanz screws. Afterwards, the distraction nuts (no. 5 in Fig. 60) are screwed up against the clamp elements to exert a low distraction force thus relieving pressure which has been placed on the intervertebral disc by the manipulation.

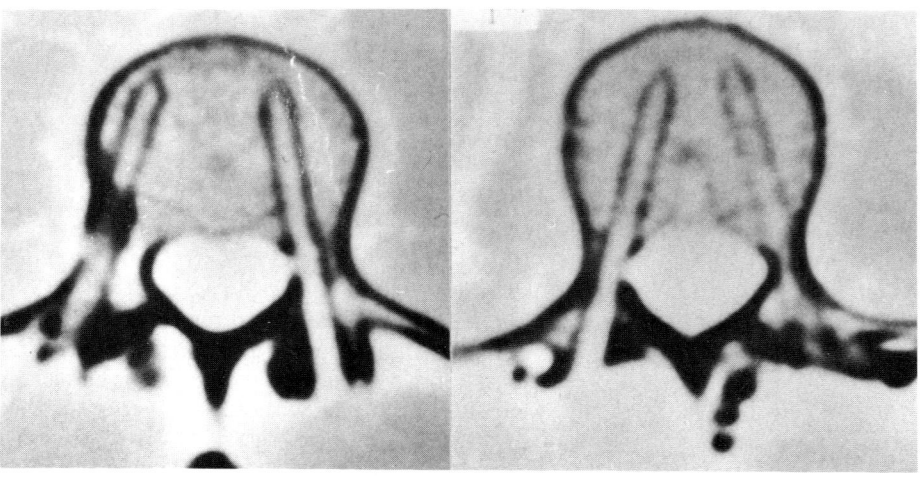

Fig. 59. Correct positioning of the Schanz screws. Their course is clearly seen for many months after implant removal.

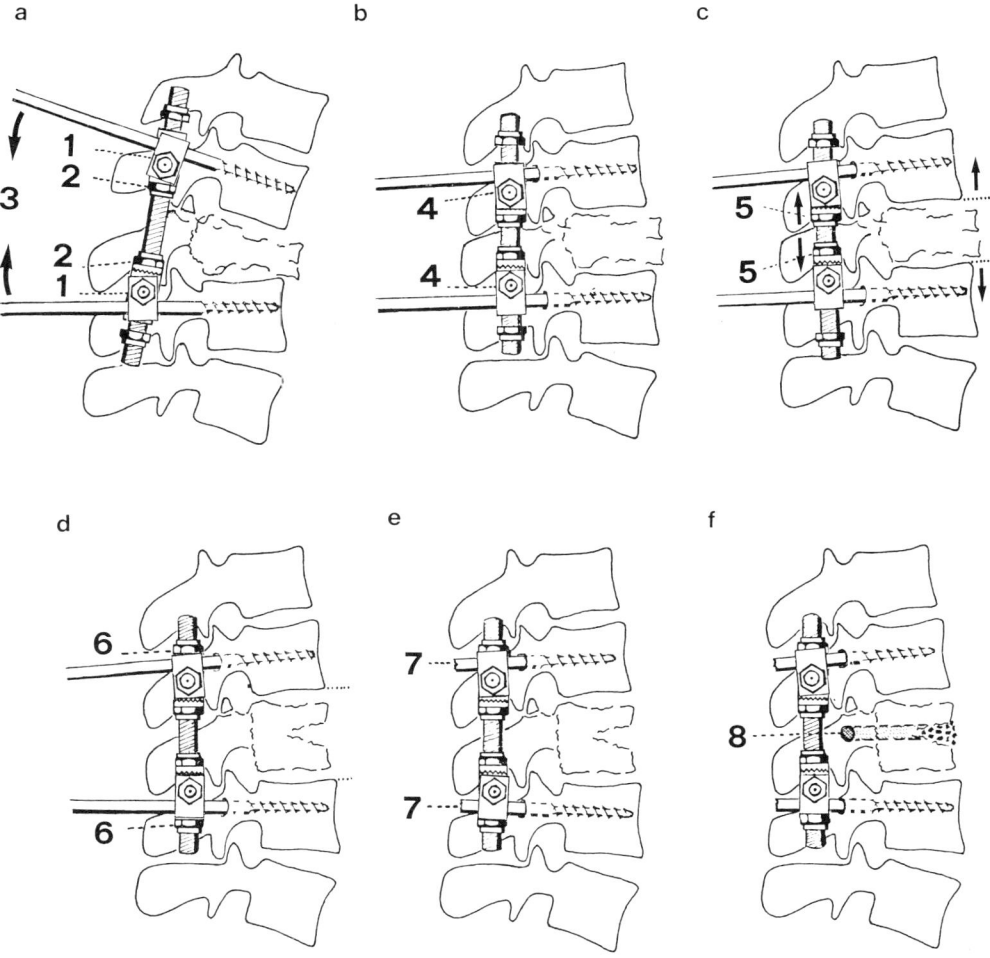

Fig. 60. Schematic representation of steps for reduction of the fracture.

a) Initially the kyphosis must always been corrected by approximating the ends of the Schanz screws (3). The lateral nuts (1) on the clamp elements are loose, the distraction nuts (2) are at a defined distance from the clamp elements or are quite loose depending on the state of the posterior wall of the vertebra (see text).
b) Tightening of the lateral nuts (4). This results in angular stability.
c) Distraction with the distraction nuts (5) in order to restore the anatomical height of the vertebra.
d) Tightening of the counter nuts (6), which results in rotational stability.
e) Removal of the projecting ends of the Schanz screws (7) with special bolt cutter.
f) Transpedicular cancellous bone grafting.

*Chance fractures [61] and pure dislocations:* In this type of fractures with destruction of the posterior columns, the fragments should be pressed together and the implants should exert a pure tension band effect where the anterior column can be subjected to pressure loading. As described above, correction of the kyphosis (or manual reduction in dislocations) is carried out with the clamps sliding freely intially, but no distraction is subsequently carried out. On the contrary, slight compression is applied from the ends of the rods with the counter nuts (no. 6 in Fig. 60).

*All other types of fracture with comminution of the posterior wall of the vertebral body:* In this group of patients (which is by far the largest in

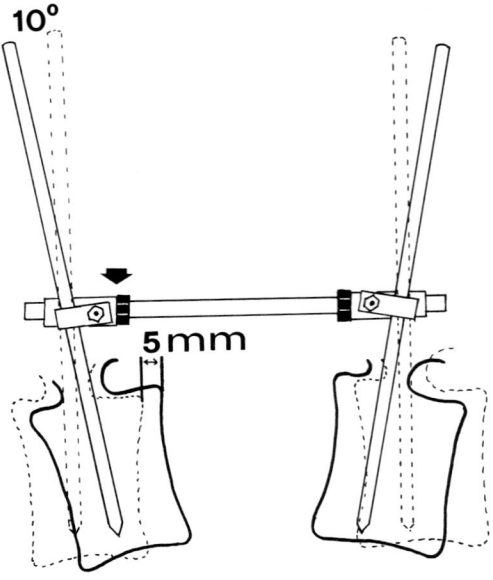

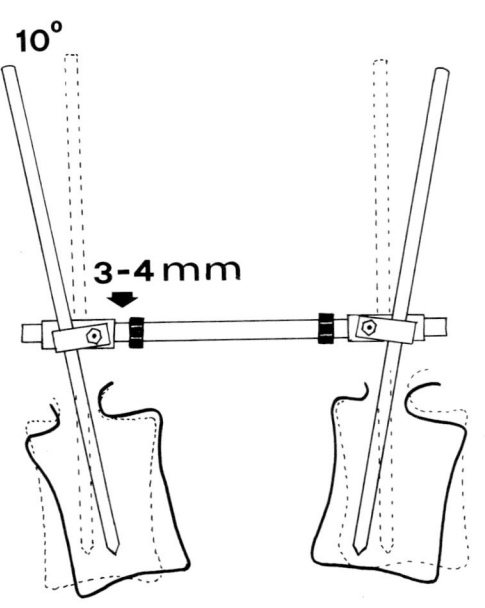

Fig. 61. Figure to show correction of kyphosis by approximating the dorsal ends of the Schanz screws. If the clamp elements are held distracted using the distraction nuts, the center of rotation for the Schanz screws is through the axis of the clamp, i.e. too far dorsally, so that correction of 10° of kyphosis results simultaneously in an increased height of the posterior edge of the vertebra by not less than 5 mm. This is not desirable. The clamp element should be able to slide 3–4 mm per 10° of kyphosis to prevent this.

number), there is a theoretical danger that fragments of the posterior wall of the vertebra may displace posteriorly into the vertebral canal during correction of the kyphosis when pressing together the ends of the Schanz screws. Thus the posterior wall of the vertebra must be protected against pressure in correcting the kyphosis. This can be achieved using the distraction nuts. If the distraction nuts touch the clamp elements before reduction of the kyphosis, the center of rotation will be displaced from the plane of the posterior edge of the vertebra to the plane of the axis of the clamp. This is demonstrated in Figure 61, showing that a distraction of at least 5 mm has taken place in the plane of the posterior wall at the same time per each 10° correction of the kyphosis. However, this amount of distraction is not possible where the ligaments are preserved, preventing an adequate correction of the kyphosis. If all the ligaments are ruptured, an undesirable over-distraction would occur. Figure 62 shows a clinical example, where the kyphosis could not be corrected because of the prior distraction. At the time of reoperation, however, the malpositioning was readily corrected by releasing the distraction nuts.

Even in this group of patients, some approximation of the clamp elements must take place. However, for each 10° correction of kyphosis, the margin of safety is 3–4 mm between the distraction nut and the clamp element as adjusted on the threaded rod before the manipulation. By doing this, slight distraction of the fractured vertebra will still take place when the kyphosis is corrected, and the vertebra will definitely not be compressed. In these cases, the force required to press together the ends of the Schanz screws is greater, and sometimes a cerclage wire is helpful. Having done this, the lateral nuts (no. 4 in Fig. 60) are also tightened up on the clamps and then distraction is achieved by using the distraction nuts until the anatomical height of the vertebra is restored. When an anatomical position has been achieved radiologically, the counter nuts (no. 6 in Fig. 60) are tightened. The mounting now has angular and rotational stability. In order to prevent late loosening of the nuts under cyclical strain, the collar of the nuts is crimped on the flattened part of the threaded rod using pliers. On the clamp elements where this safeguard is particularly important, the flat-

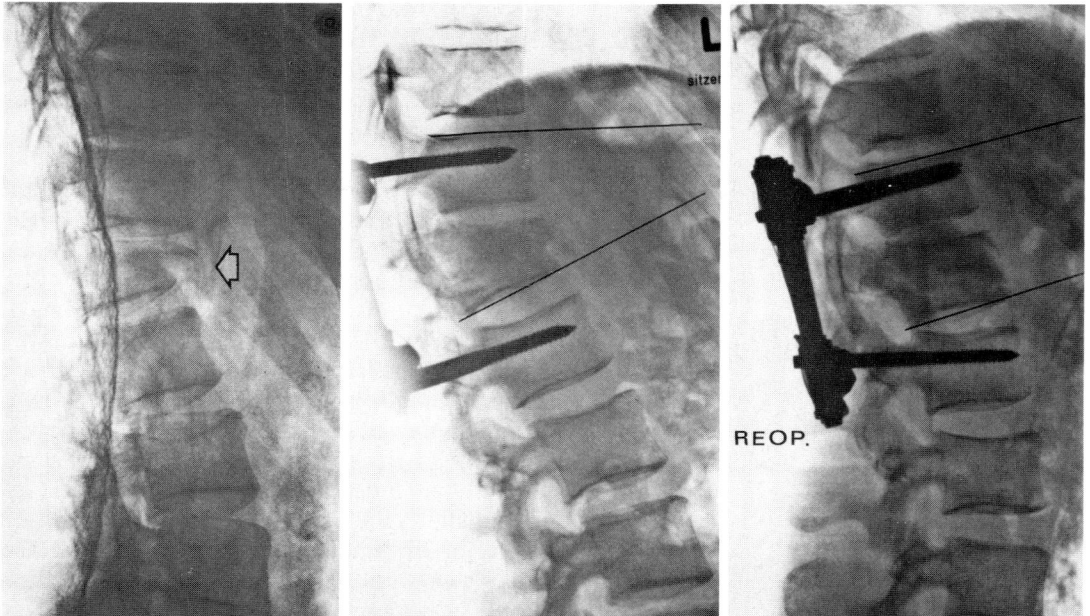

Fig. 62. At the initial operation correction of kyphosis was not successful. The mistake was initial distraction. After distraction lordosis is impossible, even applying high forces. At revision surgery three weeks later, the distraction nuts were loosened and the kyphosis could be corrected without any problem (patient K.B., male, 27 years).

tened parts of the threaded bolts are automatically in the sagittal plane. On the longitudinal rods the sagittal adjustment should be made at the beginning of the reduction as mentioned above, in order to make the procedure easier. On removal of the implant, the nuts can be loosened with a wrench despite the crimping (see Section 8.4). The dorsally projecting ends of the Schanz screws are simply cut off using special bolt cutters from the fixator instrument set (Fig. 41). These cut without a jolt and without a sharp edge as occurs when the large Harrington cutters are used. As a rule, the remaining 5 mm long ends which continue to project cause no problem. In very thin individuals, they can be screwed in deeper with special pliers even after the nuts have been tightened, provided there is enough room anteriorly between the tip of the screws and the anterior vertebral cortex. The paravertebral musculature is levered back over the rods, and wound closure does not give rise to any problems.

The internal fixator is now mounted. If a lateral dislocation is present, diagonal cerclage wires can be placed around the Schanz screws before insertion of the rods (Fig. 63). These wires improve stability against lateral tilting, but the use of the cross-linking device mentioned in Section 6.3 is safer.

The internal fixator can be inserted from T8 distally to the sacrum. In the cranial part of the thoracic spine, the pedicles become very narrow and as a rule they are not suitable for the Schanz screws. Occasionally in instrumenting the spine at lumbosacral level, the iliac wing may prevent mounting of the clamps, and some resection may be necessary using an osteotome.

A model skeleton in the operating theater helps three-dimensional conceptualization. Use of the internal fixator allows all other additional measures which may be indicated to be performed, such as removal of fragments from the spinal canal, posterolateral fusion, screw fixation of the intervertebral joints and transpedicular cancellous bone grafting. If the vertebral arch is fractured, it is not necessary to remove it unless there is some specific indication such as a dural rupture, or for removal of bony fragments. The

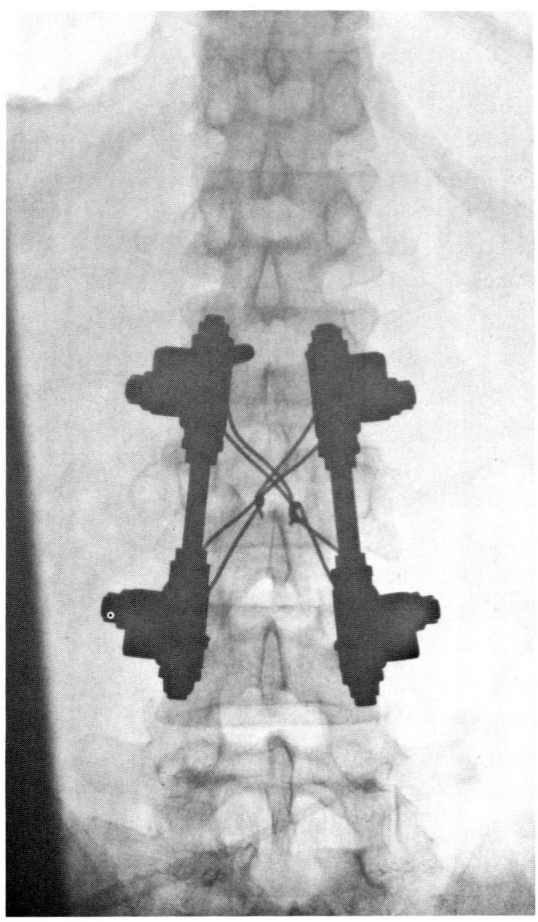

Fig. 63. Example of diagonal wiring.

implant leaves sufficient space for a postero-lateral fusion.

A prior laminectomy is not a contraindication to the use of the internal fixator. Indeed the introduction of the Schanz screws is made even more simple because the remnants of the pedicles become more easily visible. Even a previous dorsal fusion with instability does not prevent the use of the fixator, since the pedicles can always be localized using the image intensifier.

## 8.2 Anterior cancellous bone grafting

Immediate stability is ensured by the fixator. However, the long term stability is based on bony healing of the vertebral column, as no implant can hold out in the long term without fatigue.

Rapid fracture consolidation is the aim in order to obtain an anterior column capable of carrying load. In the vast majority of operatively treated fractures the vertebral body cancellous bone is compressed. This leaves a large ventral defect after reduction, and an integral part of the fixator instrumentation is the filling of ventral defects with autologous bone graft. This is possible in two ways using the posterior approach without additional anterior surgery.

DANIAUX [31, 32] described a procedure where a channel of 6 mm diameter is made into the pedicle of the fractured vertebra, the drill being directed slightly cranial to the defect. A small funnel, the wall of which must reach into the vertebral body itself to protect the vertebral canal from unintended penetration in the pedicle region, allows the transplanted bone to be pushed anteriorly into the defect (Fig. 64). Because the diameter of the funnel is small, the bone graft must be separated into very small pieces. Optimally, it should have a paste-like consistency. A well proved technique for harvesting of the graft from the upper part of the ilium is described in Section 8.3. Often a surprising amount of bone graft can be introduced into the defect. However, it is usually sufficient to place the graft from only one side. Care is taken to push the graft into the anterior part of the vertebral body not trying to fill also potential cavities in the posterior part.

Transpedicular cancellous bone grafting is best carried out once the fixator has been mounted and distraction is completed, the fragments are then held well apart. The longitudinal rod of the fixator does not prevent surgery to the pedicle of the fractured vertebra as the threaded rod lies medially due to the shape of the clamp elements.

ARNOLD [7] suggests another approach, where he performs a basal osteotomy of the transverse process of the fractured vertebra (Fig. 65). The posterolateral surface of the vertebral body is reached with blunt dissection and the cavity can be filled from here through a window. Since the route runs lateral to the pedicle, there is an increased distance to the vertebral canal which is safer. Indeed, using this technique, a bent spreader can be introduced into the vertebral body and used for reduction of the end plates.

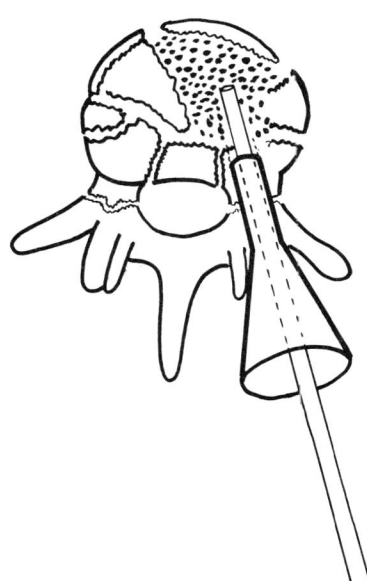

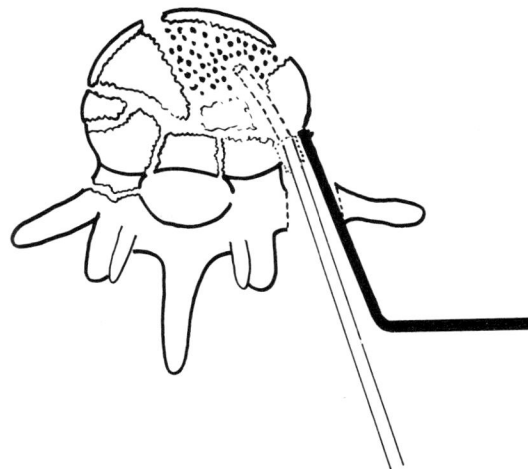

Fig. 65. Diagram to show filling of the defect in the vertebral body by osteotomy of the transverse process described by ARNOLD [7].

Fig. 64. Diagram of a transpedicular cancellous bone grafting as described by DANIAUX [32]. It is most important that the funnel reaches well into the vertebral body itself so that the bone graft cannot penetrate through a lesion of the pedicle into the vertebral canal.

## 8.3 Bone graft harvesting

The following technique has proved to be a simple, rapid and effective method for obtaining the necessary autologous bone graft material in a finely ground form (DICK [40]). Through a slightly curved skin incision just below the posterior aspect of the iliac crest and the posterior superior iliac spine, the upper part of the posterior ilium is exposed subperiosteally. With a conventional hip prosthesis acetabular reamer of 44 mm or 46 mm in diameter, bone graft can be removed and simultaneously converted into a paste-like mixture of finely ground cortical and cancellous bone. In order to facilitate the start of reaming and to avoid the reamer sliding, it is recommended that a small round window is chiseled initially in the outer cortex. By sideways movement of the reamer using the shaft, the area of removal can be extended and a very large amount of bone can be obtained. The depth of bone removed is easy to control, and the inner cortex of the pelvis remains intact. Reamers which collect the bone are most practical, but any available reamer can be used.

Hemostasis is achieved by pressing collagenous felt onto the defect surface. Redivac drainage is inserted superficial to the gluteal musculature.

The autologous bone paste obtained in this way is not only suitable for filling cavities, but for all kinds of dorsal and ventral spinal fusions, because the bone can be shaped to fit irregular surfaces closely. It also has a much larger surface area, and vascularization can take place throughout the whole grafted area simultaneously as a field phenomenon. Thus consolidation proceeds very rapidly, as demonstrated in Section 9.5 with intervertebral lumbosacral fusions.

## 8.4 Implant removal

After bony consolidation of a fracture as well as in non-traumatic cases with the exception of tumor surgery, we recommend routine removal of the internal fixator. There are three reasons for this:

– Due to the elastic properties of bone and the intervertebral disc, micromovement will continue in the implant and lead ultimately to fatigue fractures of the implant. When this occurs, the implant is no longer weight bearing and is unnecessary.

– Apart from the destroyed motion segment, often a functional motion segment has been included in the fixation, and this should be freed as soon as possible.
– There is bound to be some displacement of the paravertebral musculature by the implant, and often bursae develop around the edges of the implant. This probably accounts for the observation that even patients who were pain-free before implant removal spontaneously report that they feel «lighter» and «more mobile» after removal of the fixator.

Technically, the metal removal is not a major operation. The midline longitudinal scar is reopened and the rods are approached by sharp and blunt dissection from the midline. The screws project a few millimeters and can be exposed using Hohmann levers. Usually, the ends of the screws can be grasped with a special screw removing pliers on the instrument set, and screwed out without opening the nuts. On the inside of the clamps there are no grooves preventing this. If it is impossible to grasp the screw ends, the lateral nuts are loosened with a wrench and the fixator rods are removed. The nuts can be loosened despite the compressed collars because of the softness of the metal.

The timing of implant removal depends on the radiological consolidation, and should be carried out as soon as possible. Usually the fixator can be removed at between 9 and 12 months after instrumentation.

## 8.5 Technical difficulties

The most common cause of complications is misplacement of the Schanz screws, which must be placed with high precision so that they run correctly into the vertebral bodies in the interior of the pedicle, as shown in Figure 67.

If they are introduced too far medially, the spinal canal is breached as shown in Figure 68 in an isolated vertebral body specimen.

It is known from computer tomograms and myelograms that there is some space left between the wall of the pedicle and the nerve roots. However, it is conceivable that penetration of the vertebral canal could give rise to an epidural hemorrhage. Among our 183 patients, there has not been a single case where this happened.

If the Schanz screw is placed with too little convergence perpendicularly from the entry point described in Section 8.1, the tip can easily displace laterally and advance along the outer aspect of the vertebral body as shown in Figure 69. This may lead to a reduction in stability. One of our cases developed a secondary kyphosis of 10° where a screw had been misplaced too laterally, as described and illustrated in Section 10.2. In a second case with similar screw positioning, the fracture healed with a good result without complications, as shown in Figure 70.

The correct amount of convergence can be seen on an AP X-ray, where all four screw tips should be seen between the longitudinal rods, but should not cross over the midline. It has

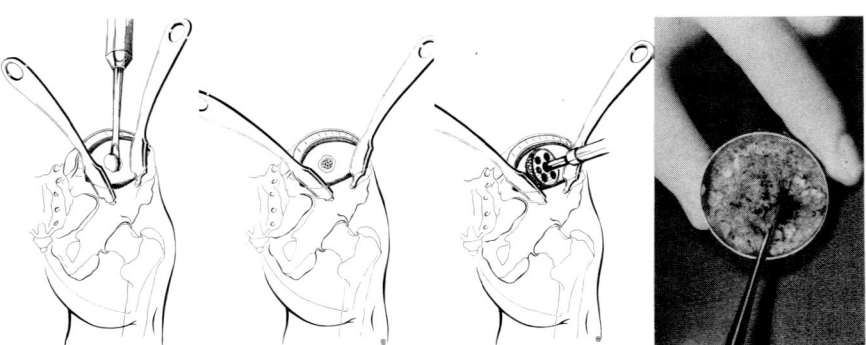

Fig. 66. Diagram of the method of bone graft retrieval. The bone is harvested in paste form using the hip prosthesis reamer as described by DICK [40]. Before reaming, it is recommended that a small window is chiseled out of the external cortical layer of the pelvis to prevent the reamer sliding off.

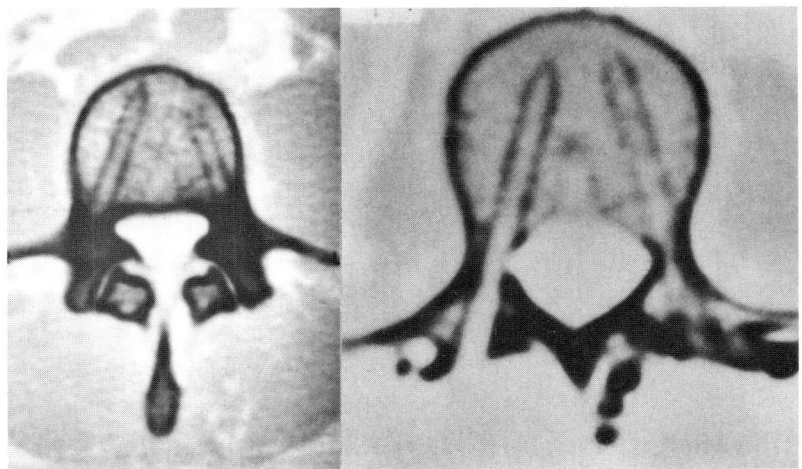

Fig. 67. Correct positioning of the Schanz screws.

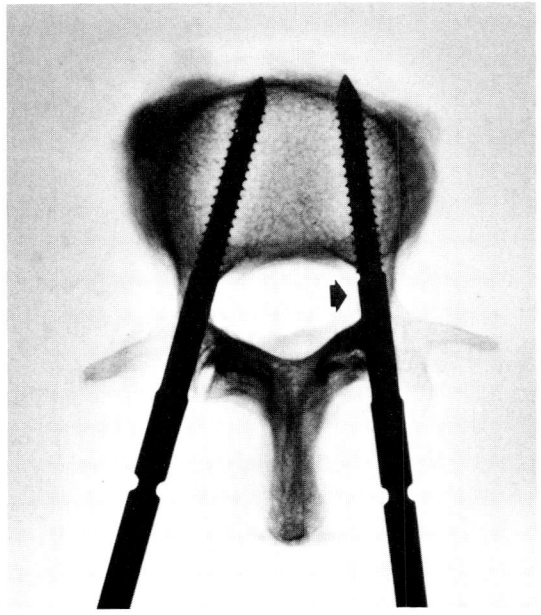

Fig. 68

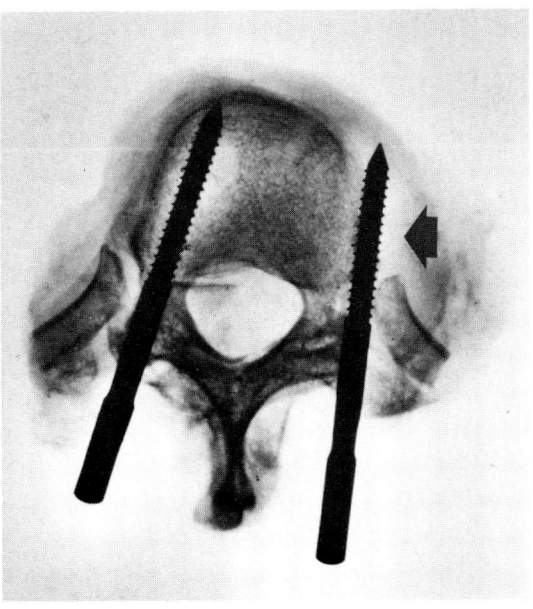

Fig. 69. Demonstration of lateral penetration of the screw due to lack of convergence.

already been mentioned in describing the surgical technique that the screw tip must never penetrate ventrally beyond the vertebra because of the danger of large vessel injury.

Another possible complication which could occur with the fixator is if the clamp is reversed by 180° so that it does not grasp properly the Schanz screw and no longer fits into the radial serration on the clamp element, as shown in Figure 72.

If the clamps need to be reversed because of an especially large or small distance between the Schanz screws, the whole clamp elements including the serrated washer should be reversed on the threaded rod as shown in Figure 73.

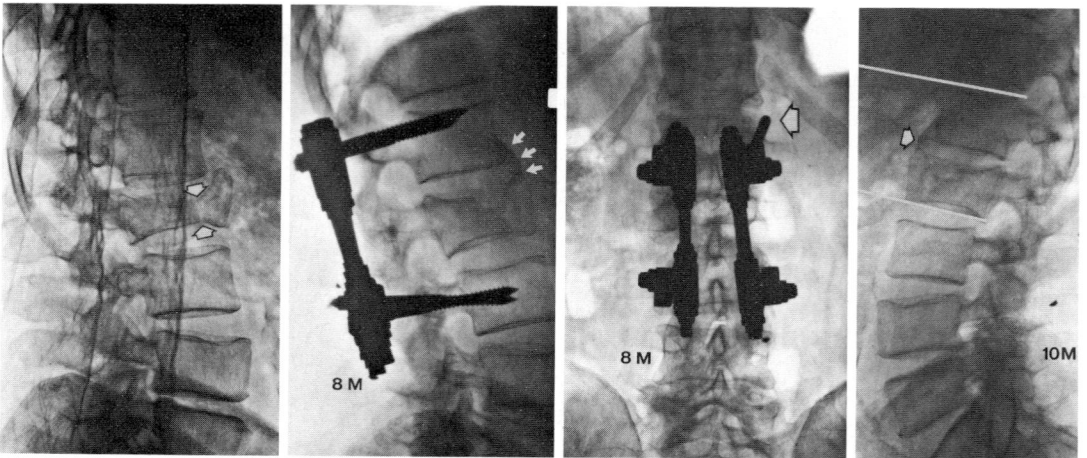

Fig. 70. One of the upper Schanz screws has penetrated laterally from the pedicle due to insufficient convergence. However, the fracture healed normally, and the reduction was maintained (patient A. W., male, 52 years old).

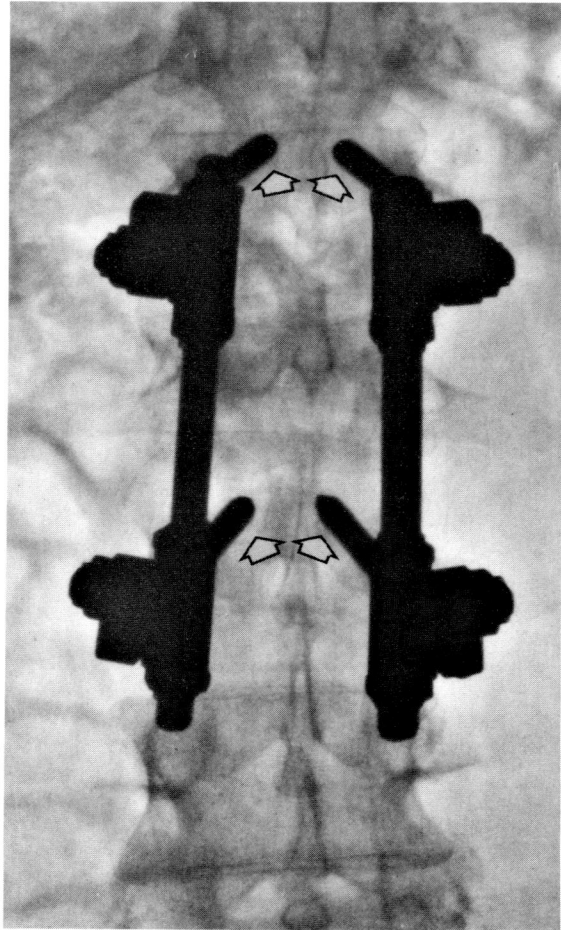

Fig. 71. On the A.P. radiograph, all four screw tips should be visible between the longitudinal threaded rods but not cross.

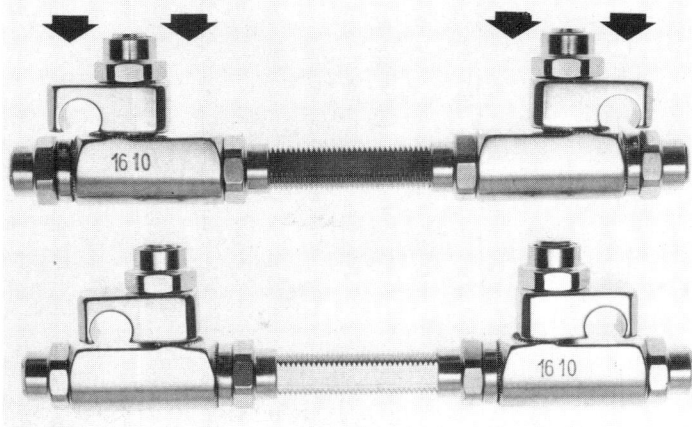

Fig. 72. The upper fixator clamps are rotated incorrectly through 180° degrees, so that the serrated surfaces no longer interdigitate.

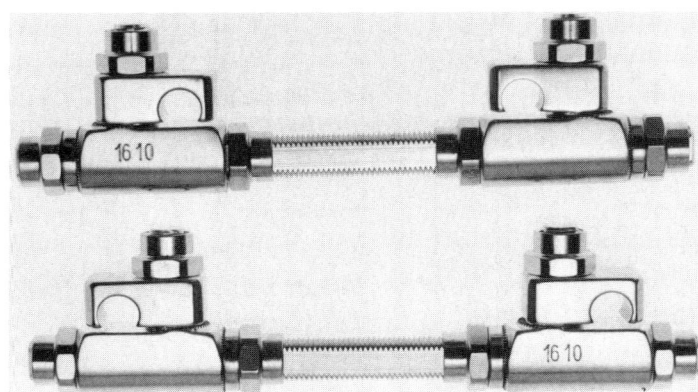

Fig. 73. The entire clamp element including the washer is correctly rotated on the threaded rod.

# 9. Applications for the internal fixator

## 9.1 Thoracolumbar and lumbar spine fractures

Fresh fractures of the spine below T8 are the main indications for the implant. It is thus suitable for the most commonly occurring types of fracture. In the upper thoracic spine where Schanz screws can only occasionally be placed due to their large size, surgical fracture treatment is much more rarely indicated. Fractures in the upper thoracic spine are also rarer in adults and are less frequently unstable. Additionally, the functional disadvantages of the long-distance rods or plates are less significant than in the lumbar spine and at the thoracolumbar junction.

The internal fixator has the following properties:

– *Short fixation distance:* The biomechanical function of the internal fixator is based on a stable angular connection between the longitudinal rods and the Schanz screws, which in turn are anchored firmly into the instrumented vertebrae so that there is no mobility at the bone-implant interface. The instrumentation hence remains restricted to the vertebrae immediately adjacent to the lesion. It thus usually only comprises three vertebrae i.e. two motion segments. It is unimportant whether these adjacent vertebrae have fractures through the posterior elements, as the Schanz screws only need to have a firm hold in the base of the pedicle and the vertebral body. In pure dislocations, monosegmental instrumentation is possible (Fig. 74).

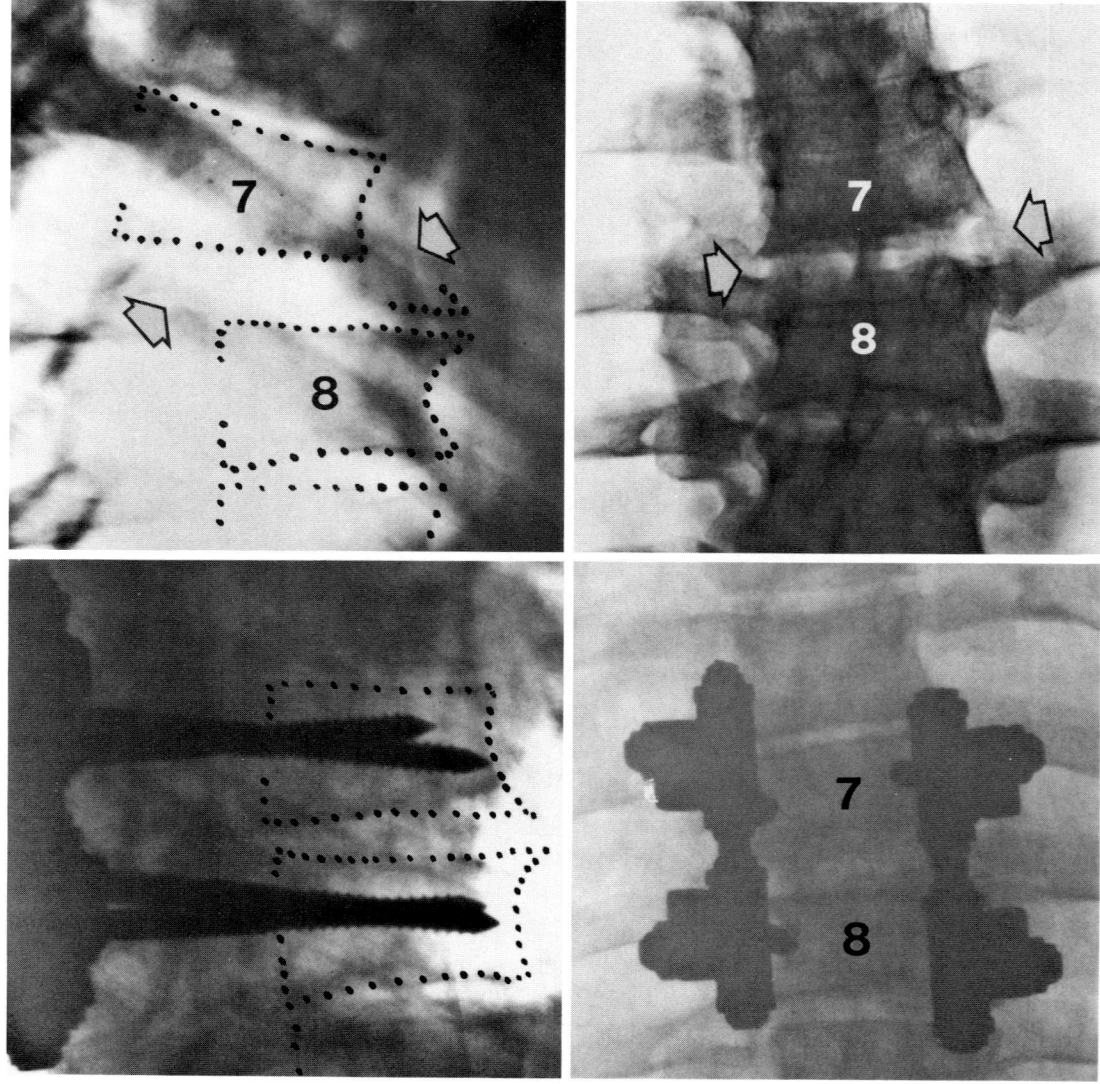

Fig. 74. In predominant disco-ligamentous lesions (dislocations), a monosegmental instrumentation may be possible (patient P.W., male, 25 years old). Fusion is mandatory in these lesions.

Five patients initially had long Harrington or Luque instrumentation, and required reoperation due to complications. Reoperation was performed by rod removal and internal fixator instrumentation. Whether the patients were paraplegic or not, all spontaneously reported a major gain in function, corresponding to the impressive radiological difference in length of the implants (Fig. 75).

If two adjacent vertebral bodies are fractured, the fixation comprises four vertebral bodies. In multiple level fractures, two separate instrumentations may be carried out, leaving a mobile segment in between.

– *Aid to reduction:* The internal fixator is not only useful as a stabilizing implant, but is also a useful instrument for fracture reduction. By means of the long lever arms of the Schanz

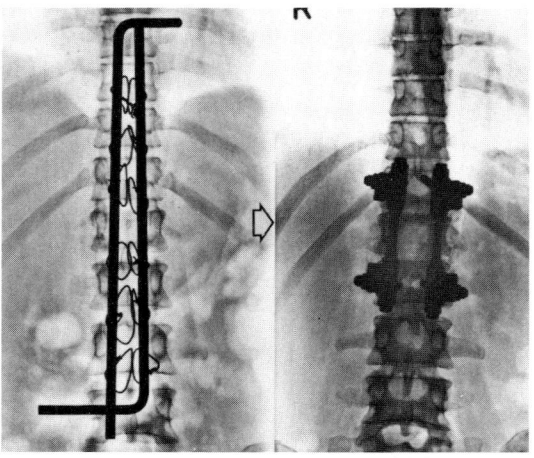

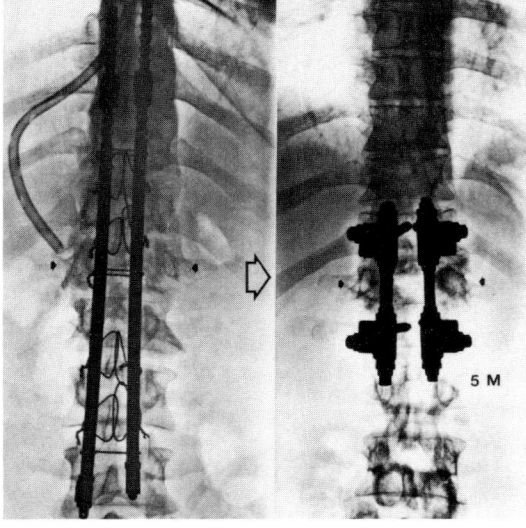

Fig. 75. Examples of the different lengths of fixation in patients whose implants were changed to an internal fixator because of complications (top, patient P.A., female, 18 years old, bottom, patient Z.A., male, 23 years old).

vertebral fractures which project into the vertebral canal similarly frequently reduce once the kyphosis is corrected and longitudinal traction applied. However, this only occurs when surgery is undertaken in the first five to ten days after the trauma. There is always some doubt that the cross-section of the vertebral canal can be restored in this way, but this can be demonstrated unequivocally using computerized tomography or myelotomography (Figs. 79, 80).

However, canal restoration cannot always been achieved, and it is therefore recommended that myelography or ultrasonography is carried out intraoperatively if there is any doubt. If continued narrowing of the vertebral canal is shown, a laminectomy should be performed and the fragments should be impacted or extracted, especially in the region of the conus.

An alternative to laminectomy for those cases is an additional anterior approach with anterior decompression and bone grafting. This can be performed without an anterior implant thanks to the stability of the fixator.

It is of utmost importance to restore the cross-sectional shape of the vertebral canal in patients with incomplete neurological injuries. In patients without neurological deficit and in patients with complete paraplegia without sacral sparing despite return of bulbocavernous reflex, the importance of this is not so great, and it is to some extent the decision of the surgeon.

Scoliotic deformities occurring in the sagittal plane can also be reduced by distraction greater on one side than on the other.

In fractures with displaced posterior wall fragments which are three or four weeks old, anterior decompression and stabilization are recommended, as there is little prospect of spontaneous reduction of the fragments by ligamentotaxis [91, 99].

screws, the position of the vertebrae can be adjusted directly in three dimensions. The thread of the longitudinal rods also gives precise control to the amount of distraction or compression applied.

Vertebral canal narrowing secondary to subluxation or kyphosis in the area of the fracture is usually corrected by reduction of the fracture. Posterior wall fragments of comminuted

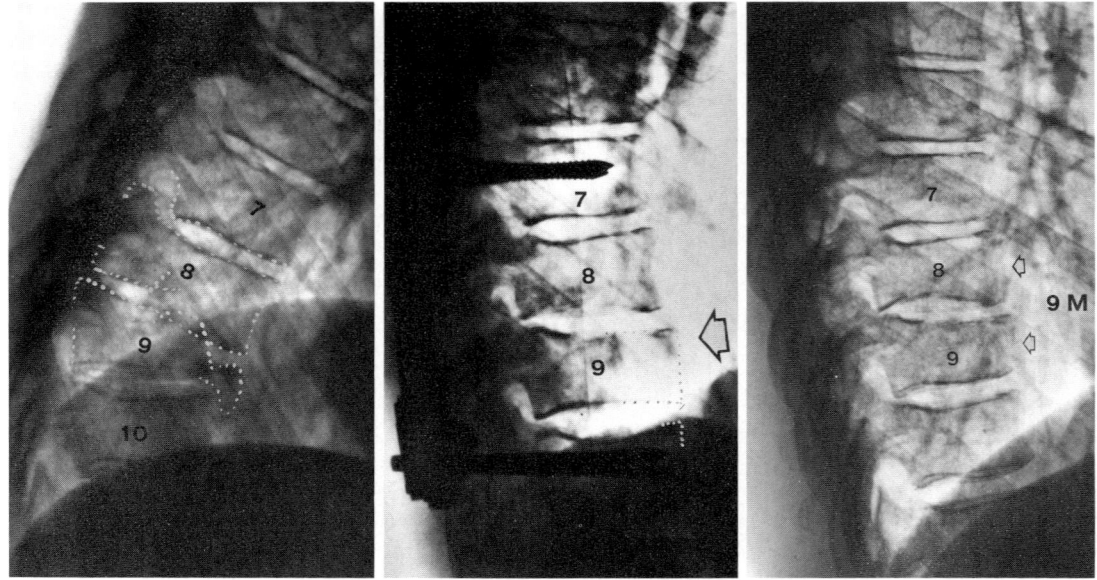

Fig. 76. In injuries of two adjacent vertebral bodies, both are bridged by the implant (patient, W. D., male, 22 years old).

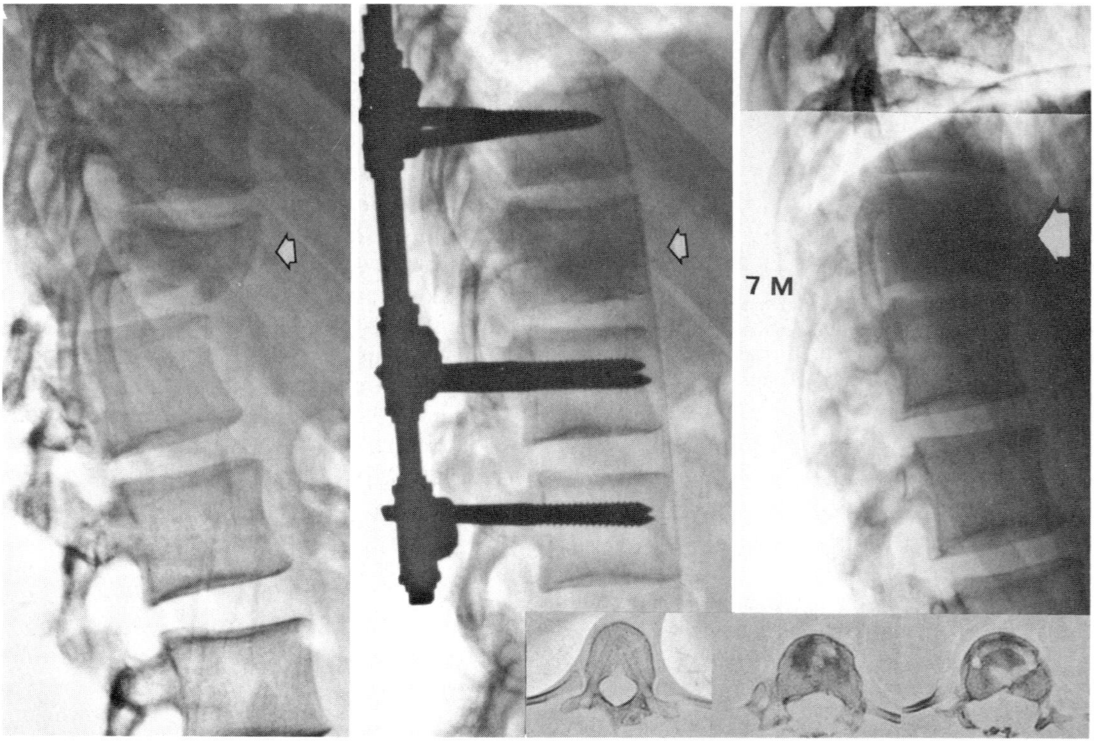

Fig. 77. Here, a lesion of the posterior elements of L1/2 was present as well as a burst fracture of T12, so that the fixator crossed both injuries. Transpedicular cancellous bone grafting was performed at T12. No fusion was performed, and the fixator was removed early to increase mobility (patient M.S., male, 25 years old).

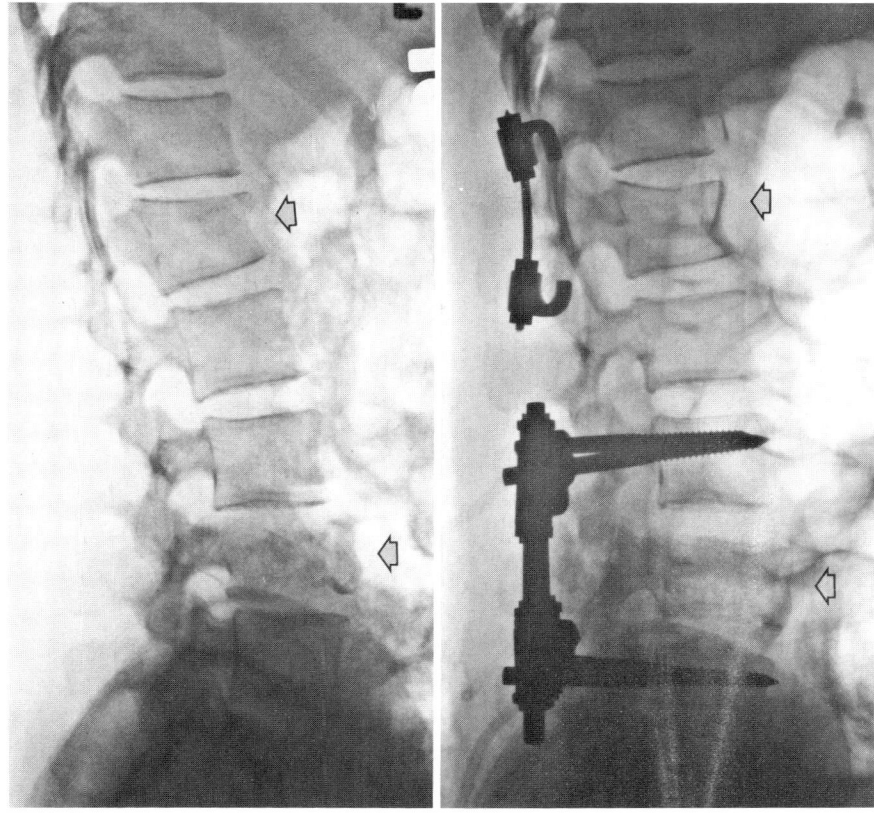

Fig. 78.
Several vertebrae
are fractured, and
separate
instrumentations
are performed
(patient, D.C.,
female,
19 years old).

– *Independence of type of fracture:* Since the internal fixator is intrinsically stable, it is equally applicable to any type of injury. It is not important whether some or all ligament connections are ruptured, whether the dorsal elements are fractured or whether the posterior wall can carry weight or not. A prior extensive laminectomy as is encountered from time to time in patients referred from other centers does not prevent instrumentation using the internal fixator, which provides the same results as in cases where it is used primarily (Fig. 83 shows such an example).

The technique of reduction for individual types of injuries is described in Section 8.1.

– *Preservation of the physiological lumbar lordosis.* As already described, distraction rods in the lumbar spine lead to an iatrogenic loss of lordosis [73], unless the kind of rod allows contouring into lordosis. However, even with these systems, it is not always possible to preserve the lordosis using distraction rods,

for example in fractures of the fifth lumbar vertebral body, because no two point fixation can be attained distally.

However, the desired lordosis can be attained over the entire lumbar spine down to the sacrum using the internal fixator.

– *Simple followup treatment.* Over the last four years, we have confirmed clinically that the instrumentation is sufficiently stable to allow early mobilization of patients. They are allowed to ambulate at three to five days, and paraplegic patients are allowed into a wheelchair after one or two weeks. Full contact corsets or plaster corsets are never necessary, and the patients wear a light three-point corset of the Jewett type for eight weeks.

When the internal fixator is used as a pure tension band with dorsal compression (chance fractures, dislocations), followup treatment is possible without any external support. In reliable and co-operative patients, we have also allowed mobilization in other types of fractures without a corset.

79

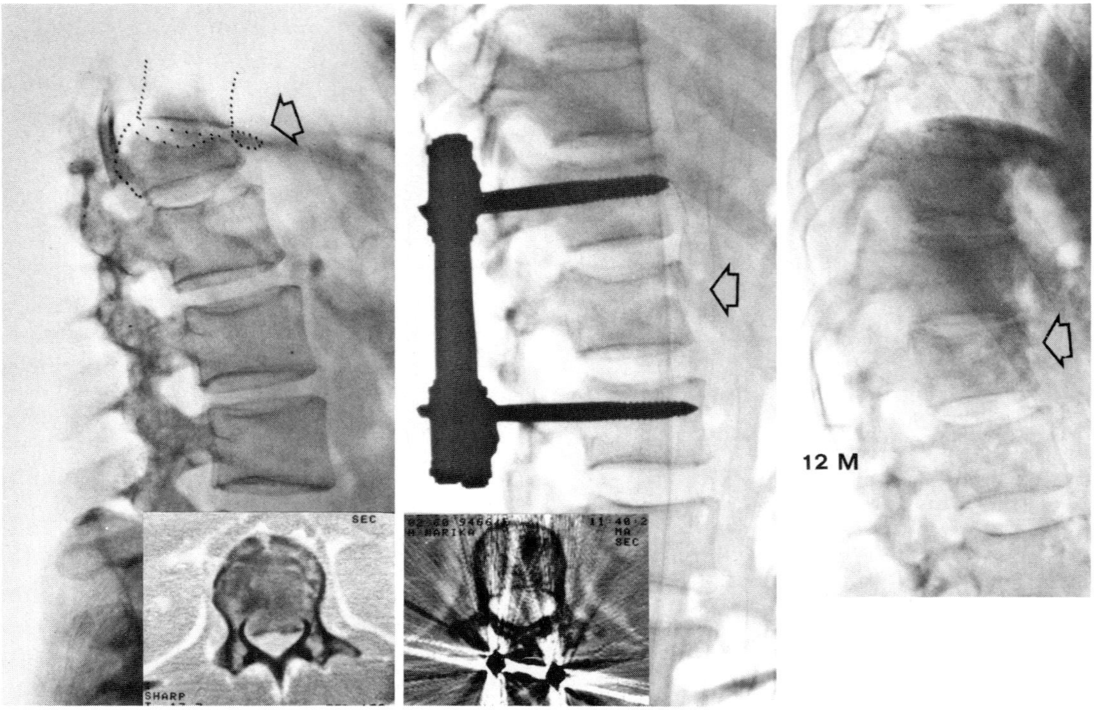

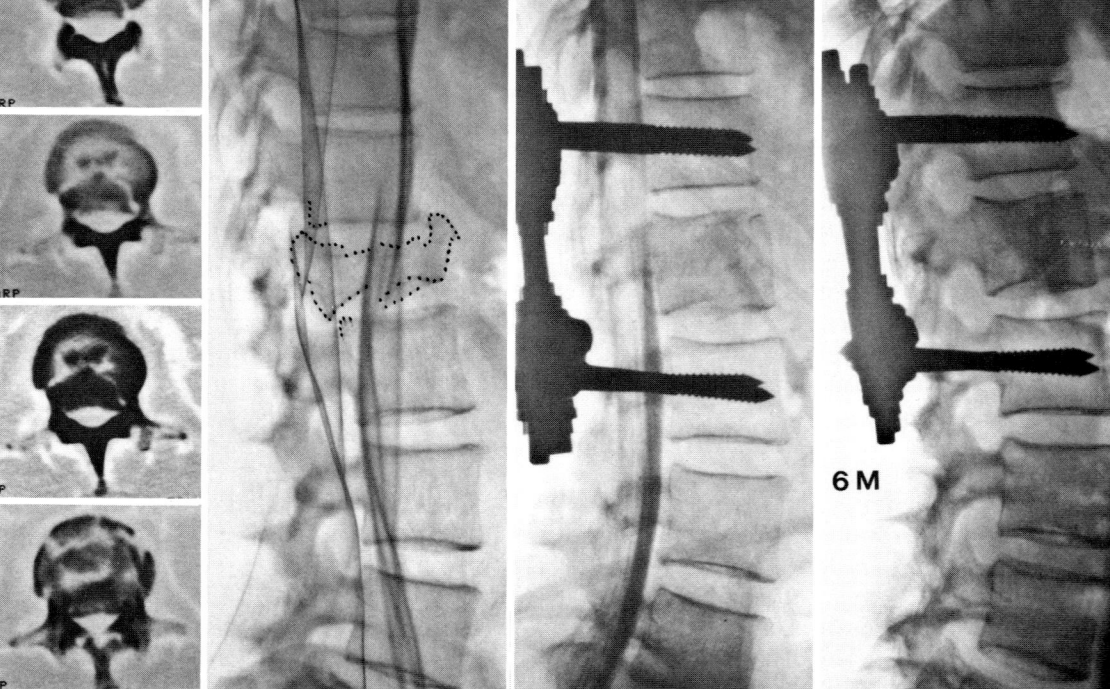

12 M

6 M

◁ Fig.79. The posterior wall of the vertebral body has been reduced merely by correcting the kyphosis and subsequent distraction, without any additional measures, as documented by CT (patient T.M., female, 25 years old, operation on the day of injury).

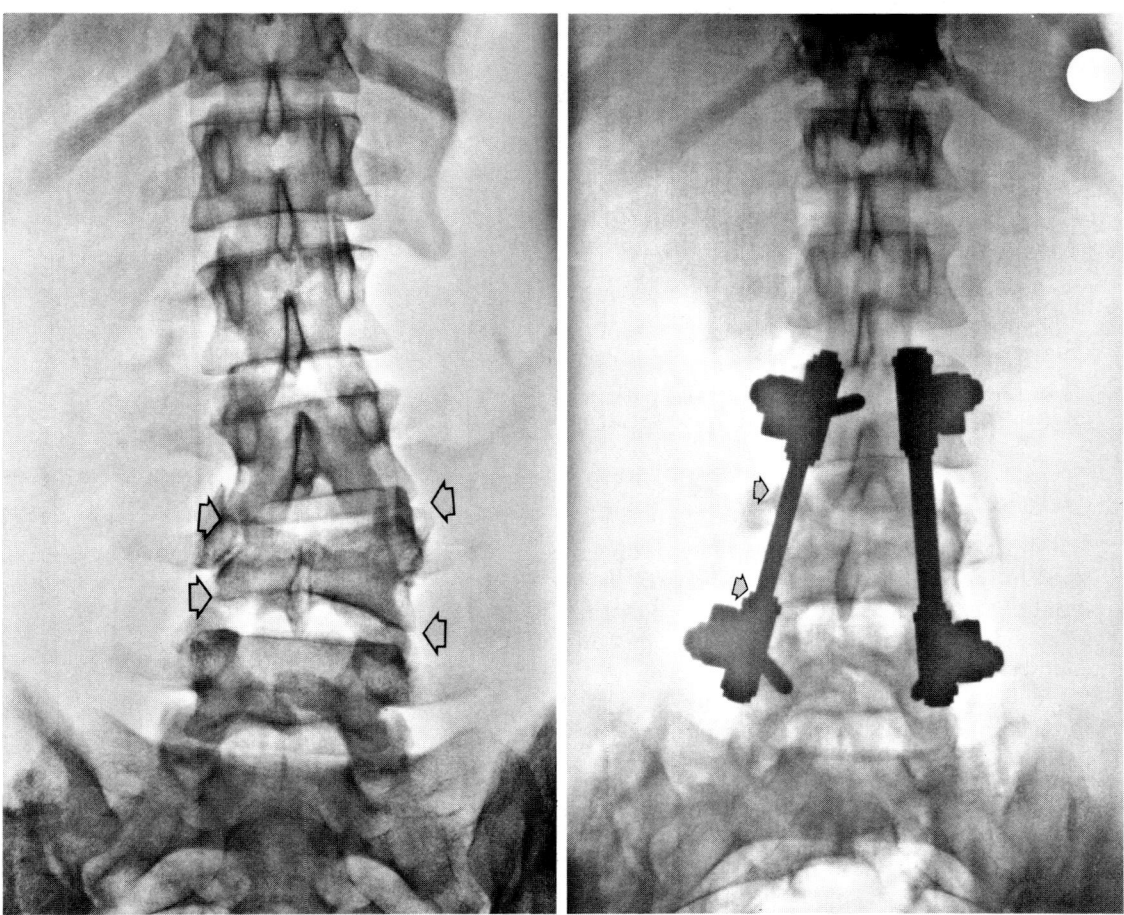

Fig. 81. Lateral deformities in the region of the fracture are corrected at the same time as correction of the kyphosis (patient W.R., female, 24 years old).

◁ Fig.80. Reduction of the fracture using the internal fixator as described without laminectomy. The myelo-tomography confirms anatomical reduction (patient C.R., female 35 years old). Transpedicular bone grafting has been performed.

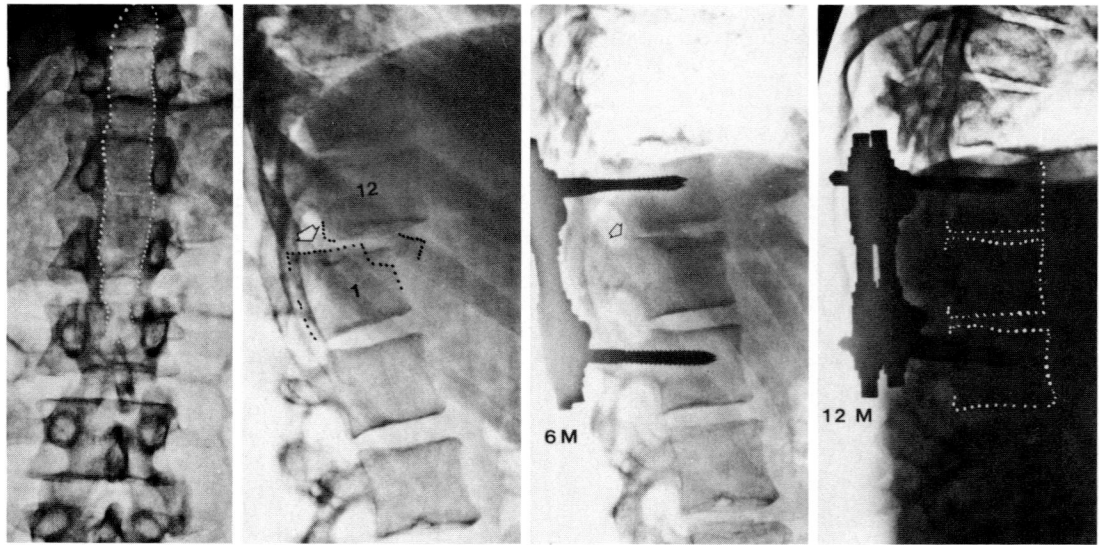

Fig. 82. Treatment of patient referred following wide laminectomy T10/L3, but with a continuing dislocation at T12/L1. Reduction fixation as for fresh fractures (patient P.M., male, 36 years old).

It must be repeated that the implant only ensures immediate stability, that the long term stability depends on bony healing, and that defects need to be filled with autologous bone as described in Section 8.2.

Figures 83–87 show typical reduction X-rays and healing in different types of fractures.

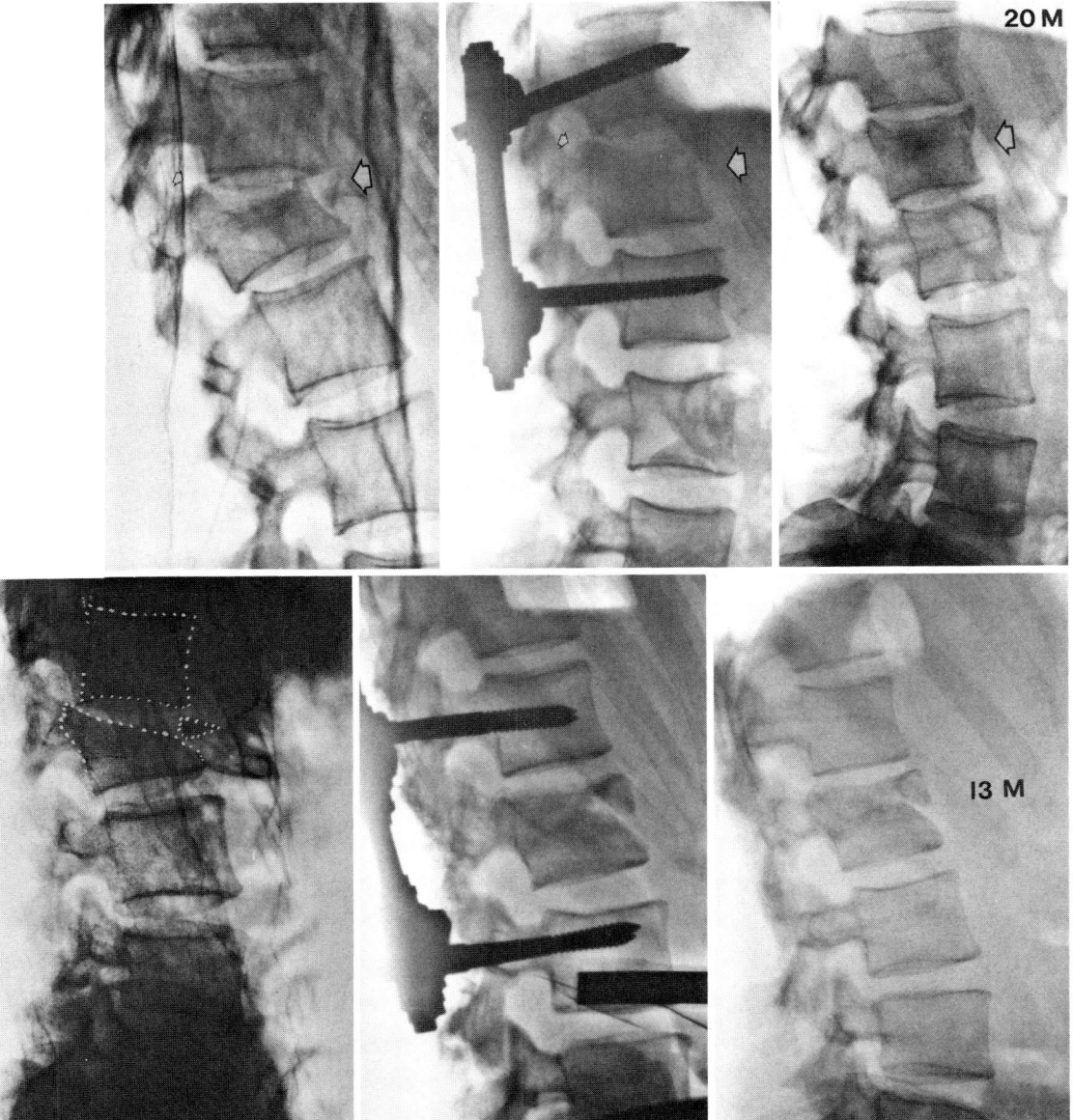

Fig. 83. Typical instrumentations in fractures. (Top, patient S.M., female, 38 years old. Bottom, patient S.A., female, 22 years old).

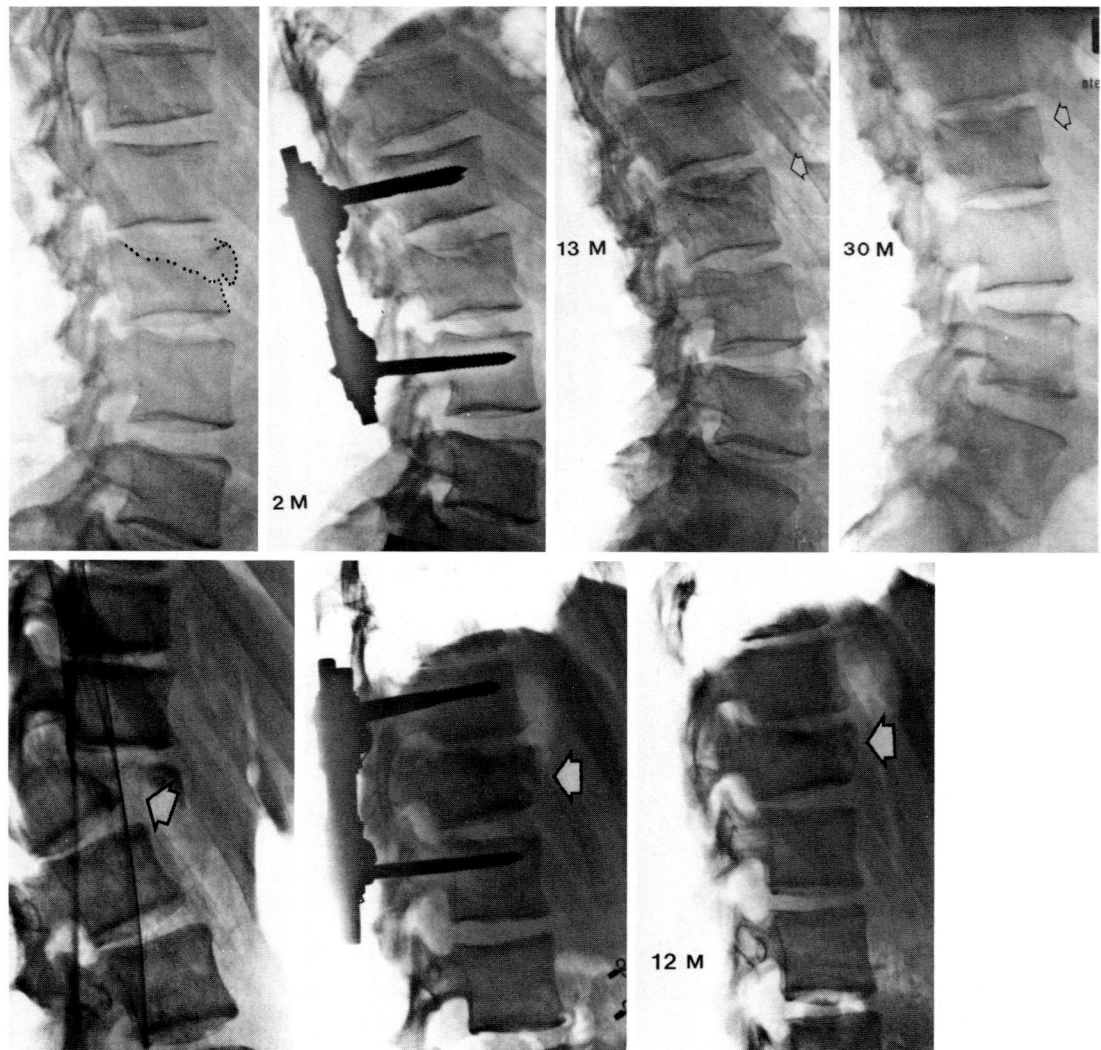

Fig. 84. Typical instrumentations in fractures. (Top, patient S. K., male, 36 years old. Bottom, patient S. J., female, 16 years old).

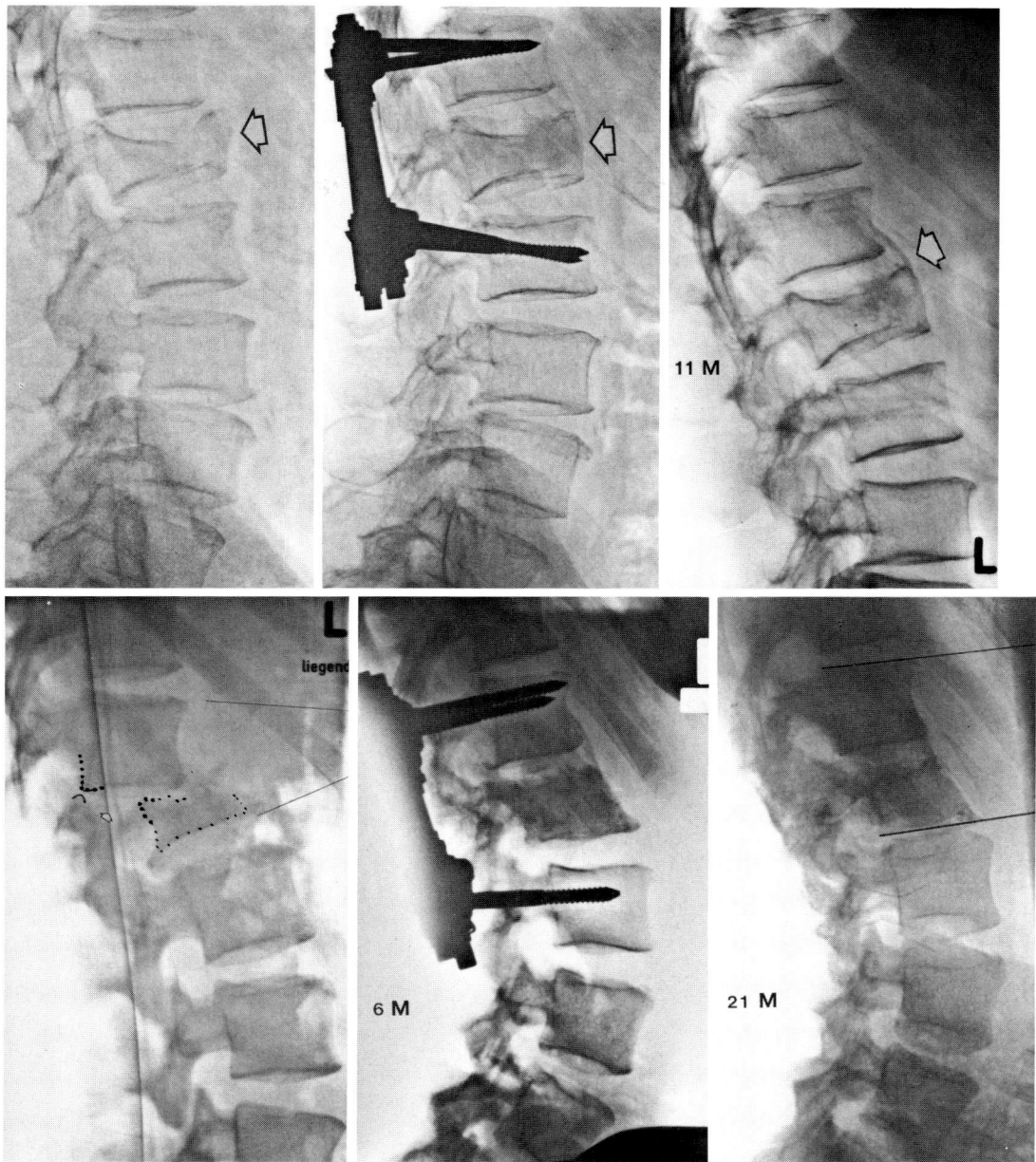

Fig. 85. Typical instrumentations in fractures. (Top, patient R. W., male, 55 years old. Bottom, patient S. E., female, 19 years old).

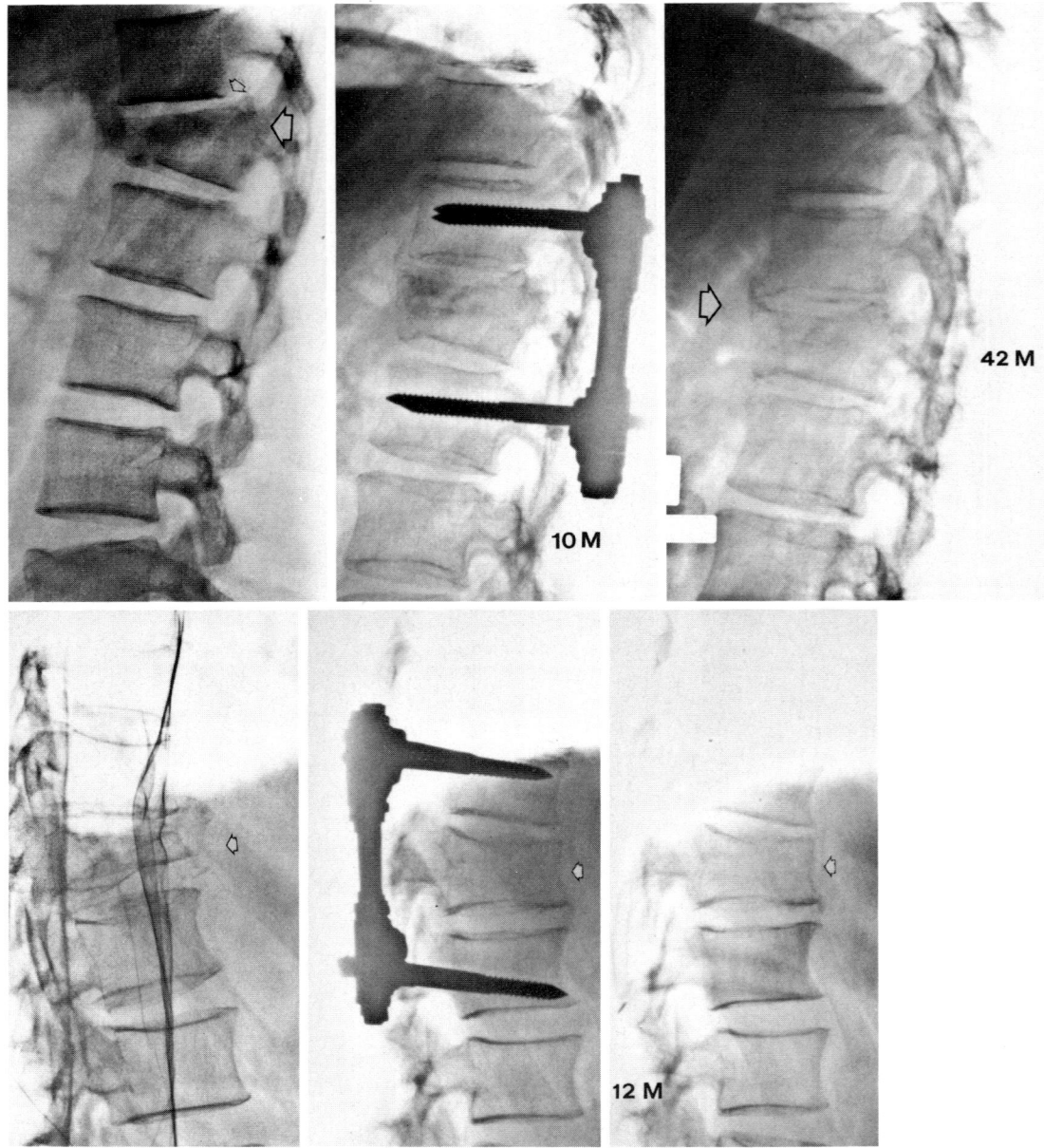

Fig. 86. Typical instrumentations in fractures. (Top, patient M.B., male, 36 years old. Bottom, patient F.J., male, 35 years old).

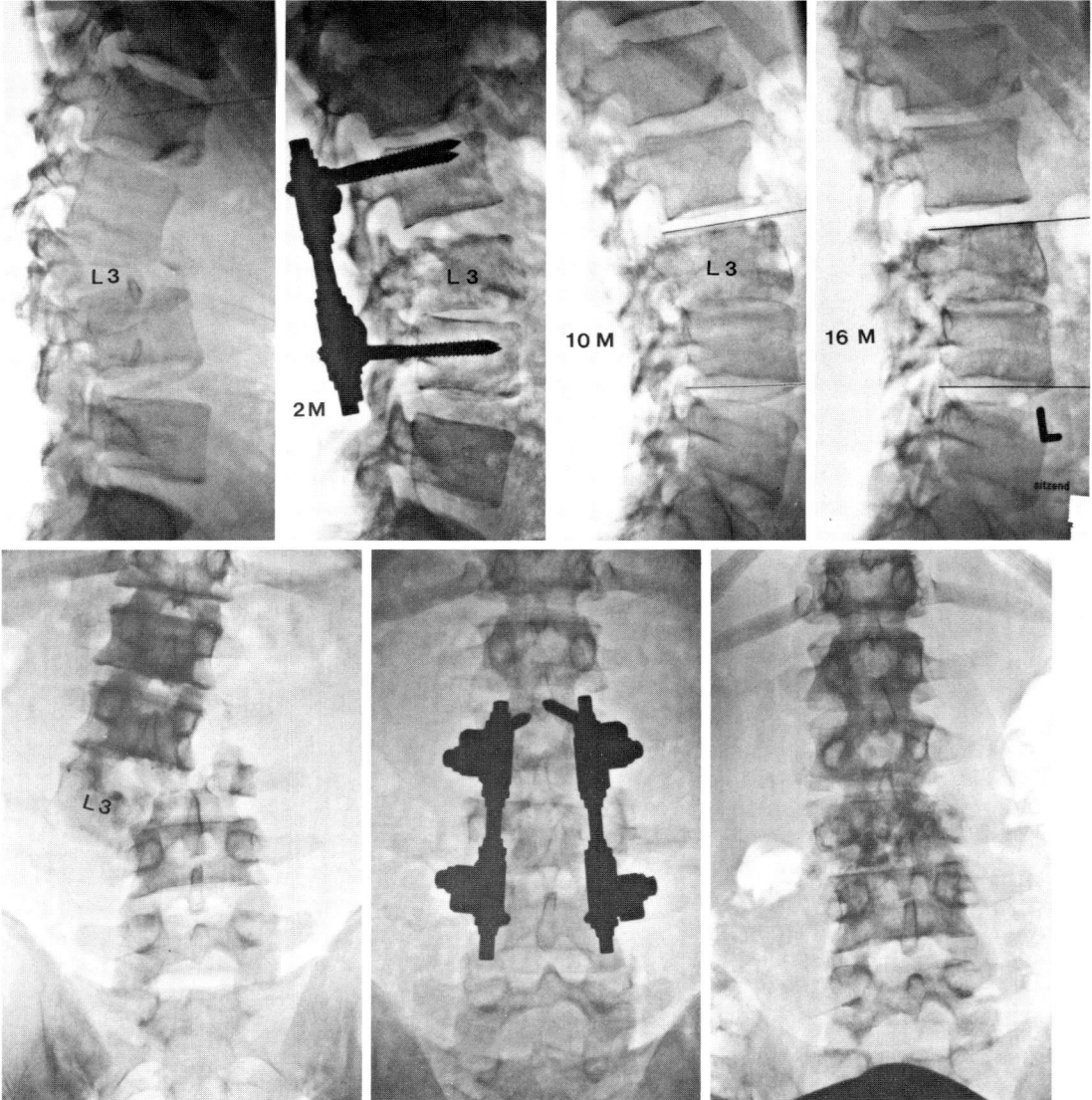

Fig. 87. Typical instrumentation in L 3 fracture dislocation. A monosegmental fusion results in a physiological lumbar lordosis. Removal of the fixator after 10 months. No late kyphosis (patient A. A., male, 21 years old).

## 9.2 Posttraumatic deformities

Some posttraumatic kyphoses can be adequately corrected by anterior spine osteotomy. In these cases, simple bone grafting is performed in the intervertebral space with a cortical bone graft (Fig. 5), or an anterior rod system may be added. Whatever the treatment, postoperative management for several months in a corset is necessary.

However, in cases where corrective osteotomy is not possible because the dorsal elements which were also fractured originally have consolidated in a malposition, or where a spondylodesis has developed, an additional posterior osteotomy may be necessary. The internal fixator has proved to be helpful here. The long lever arms of the Schanz screws allow high lordotic forces to be applied for the correction. The clamp elements on the threaded rods must be able to slide freely. Reduction is carried out using the healed posterior wall of the vertebral body as a lever. A further advantage is that followup treatment is simplified. The fixator is employed as a type of tension band and allows immediate mobilization without a corset, or with a light three-point corset.

Two examples of such late kyphoses are shown in Figures 88 and 89.

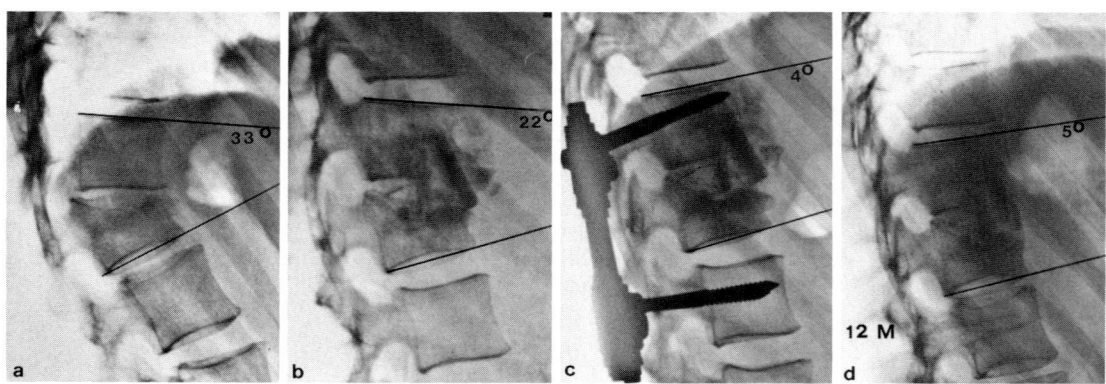

Fig. 88. Combined anterior/posterior corrective osteotomy in a posttraumatic kyphosis one year after injury. Initial procedure anterior, with a crucial gain of correction only after posterior instrumentation. Implant removal one year later (patient S.C., female, 27 years old).

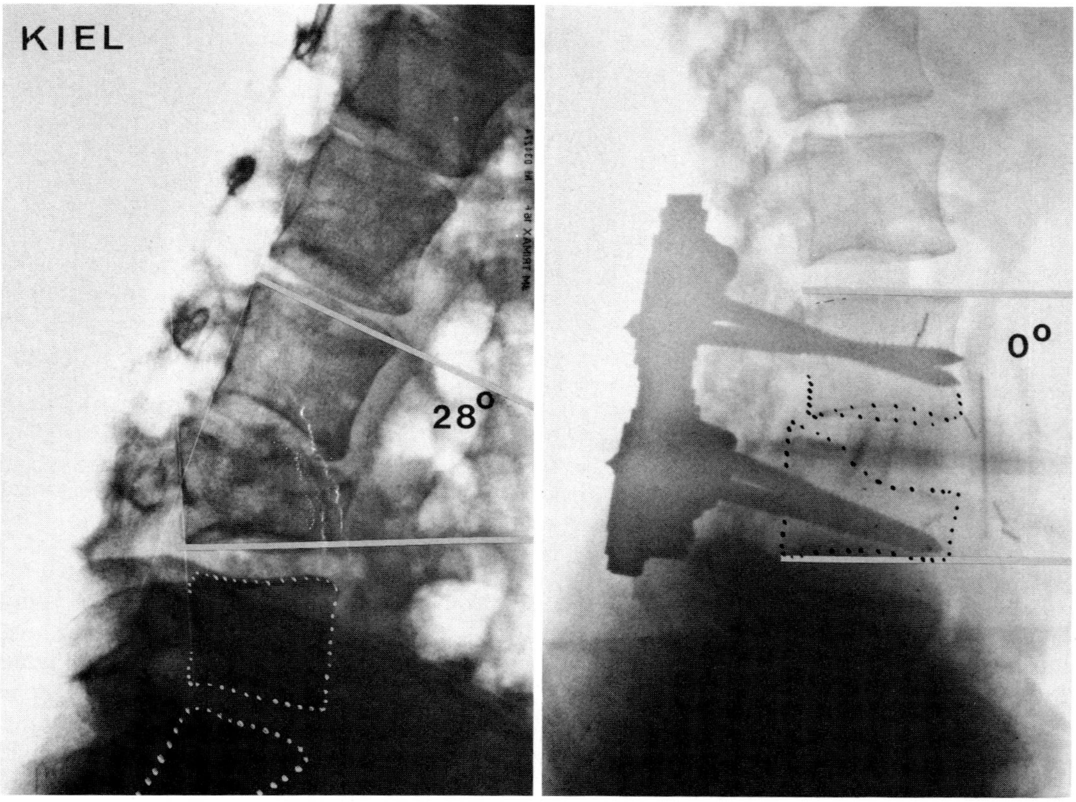

Fig. 89. Combined anterior and posterior correction of kyphosis. Since the Schanz screws have plenty of space in the wedged vertebra, the fixation can be purely monosegmental (patient L.U., female, 33 years old). By courtesy of Prof. BLAUTH, Kiel.

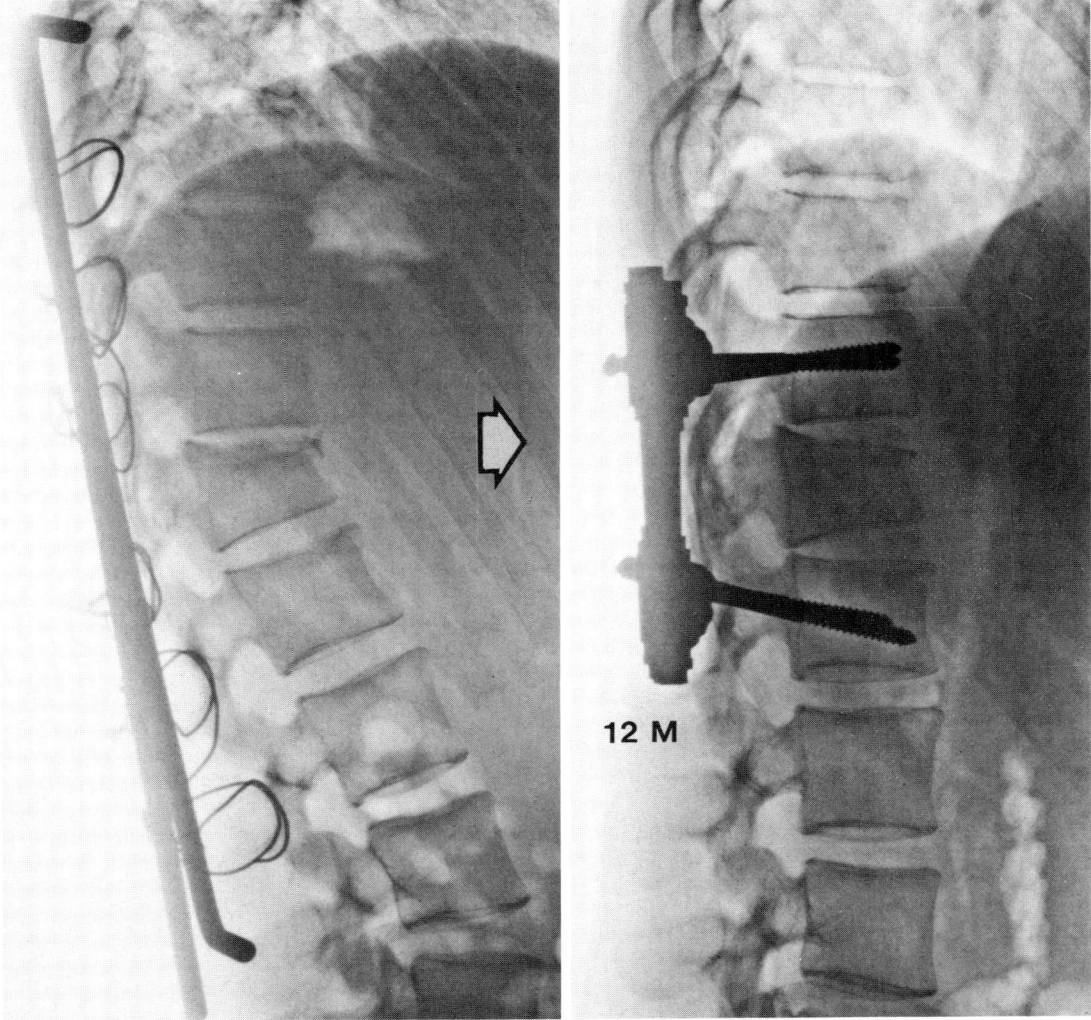

Fig. 90. Five months after Luque instrumentation, further kyphosis after breaking of the Luque wires and projection of the ends of the rods with pain. Reinstrumentation with the internal fixator. Correction was possible by posterior approach, but of course the correction only occurred at the intervertebral disc space. Posterolateral fusion. (patient P. A., female, 27 years old).

In patients with failed posterior implants, where operation must begin anyway dorsally, or in patients with permanent ligamentous instability, the fixator applied dorsally is often sufficient to reach the desired correction without anterior release (Fig. 90). It has to be completed by a posterolateral fusion.

## 9.3 Vertebral tumors and metastases

The indications for surgery in this group of patients was discussed in Section 3.3. Unfortunately, it is not uncommon that surgery is merely a way of making nursing easier and reducing pain in the last months or weeks where there are extensive metastases. In cases where there are diffuse metastases which have largely destroyed the spine, it may be difficult to find suitable anchor-

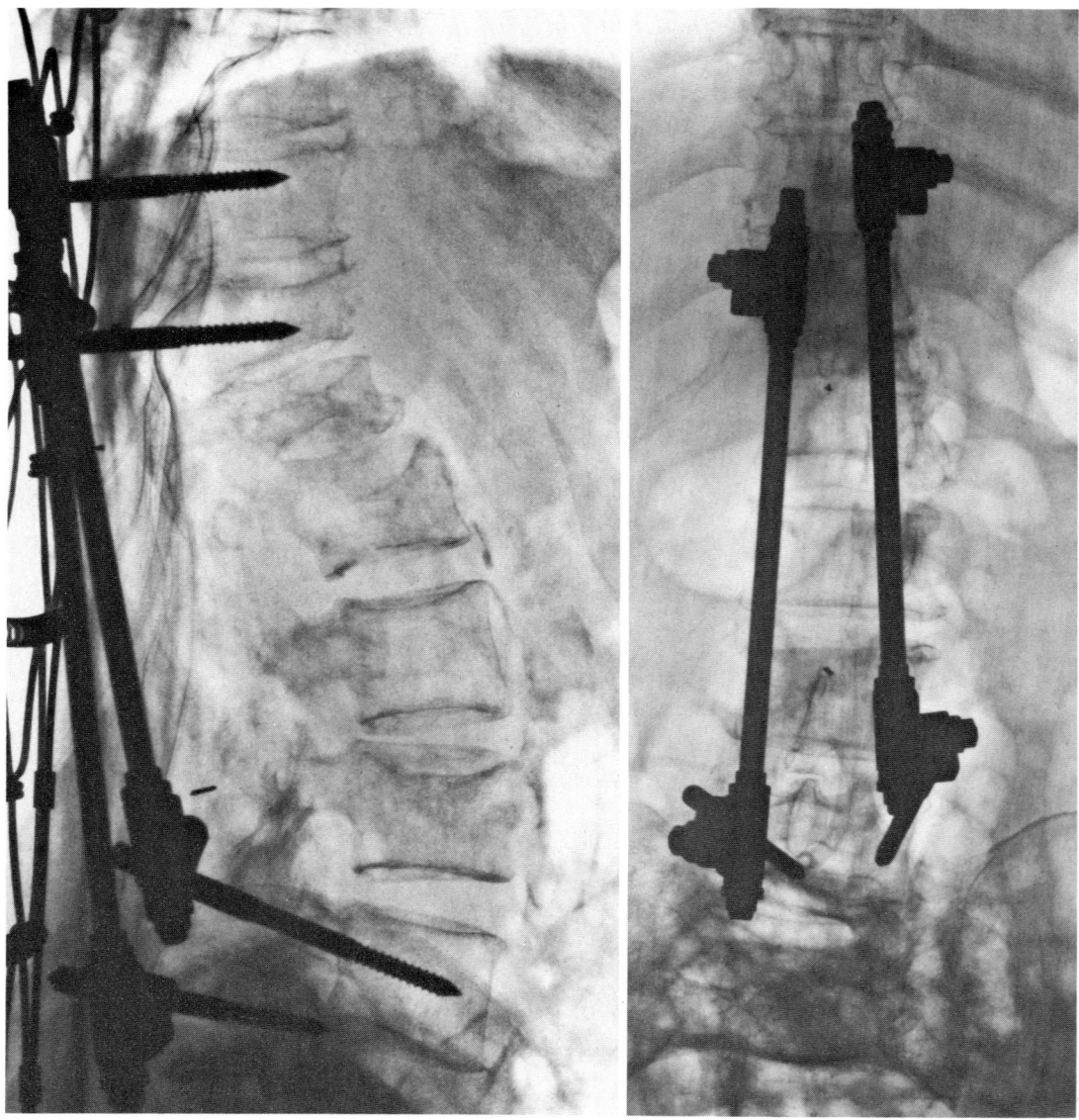

Fig. 91. Almost complete destruction of the lumbar spine due to diffuse metastatic carcinoma of the breast. After instrumentation nursing was made much easier for the five remaining months of life. The patient was able to be nursed intermittently in an arm chair (patient H.C., female, 62 years old).

ing points for the implant as shown in Figure 91. Here, the transpedicular screws can be placed away from the most severely affected area to find sufficient purchase. The threaded rods then are cut individually to length.

The internal fixator may also be suitable in certain cases where a metastasis has been treated by a laminectomy soon after the appearance of neurological symptoms, with or without tumor resection. Figure 92 shows a case where a bronchial carcinoma metastasis was resected using a costotransversectomy, and the internal fixator with its immediate stability and short fixation distance was appropriate. The patient survived for seven months without cord compression.

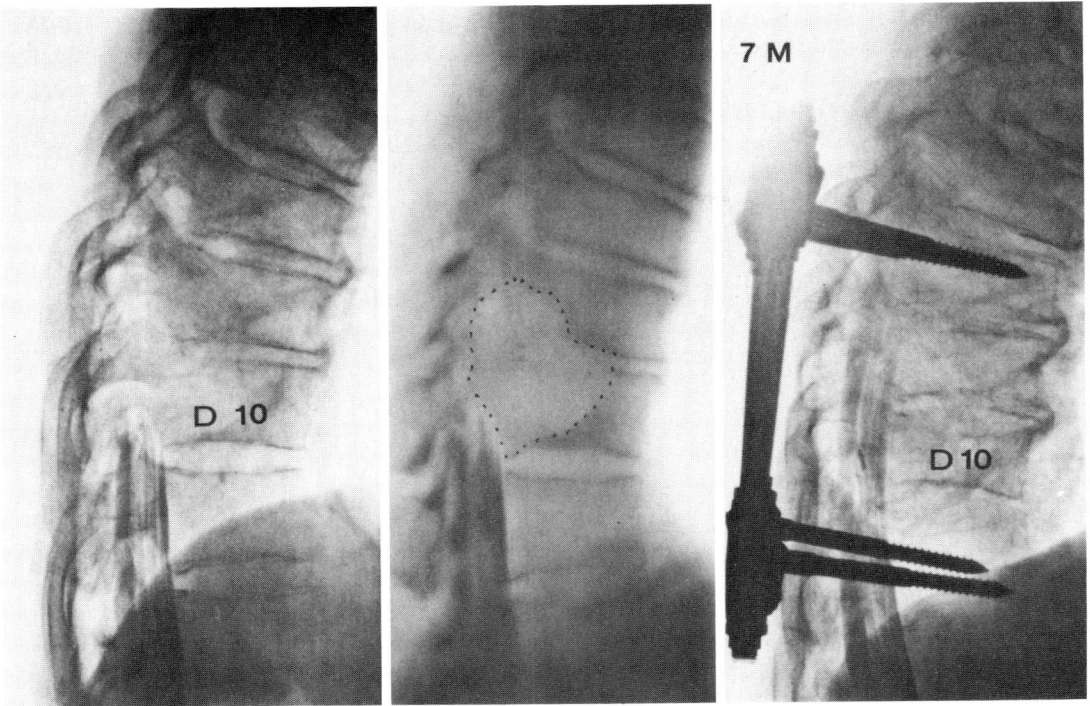

Fig. 92. Metastasis due to carcinoma of the bronchus, excised by costotransversectomy, and fused with a fixator from T8–11. The patient was free from symptoms for seven months. Subsequently he developed new symptoms secondary to a more proximal compression, when a myelogram showed the vertebral canal still patent at T9–10. He survived nine months postoperatively (patient J.N., male, 58 years old).

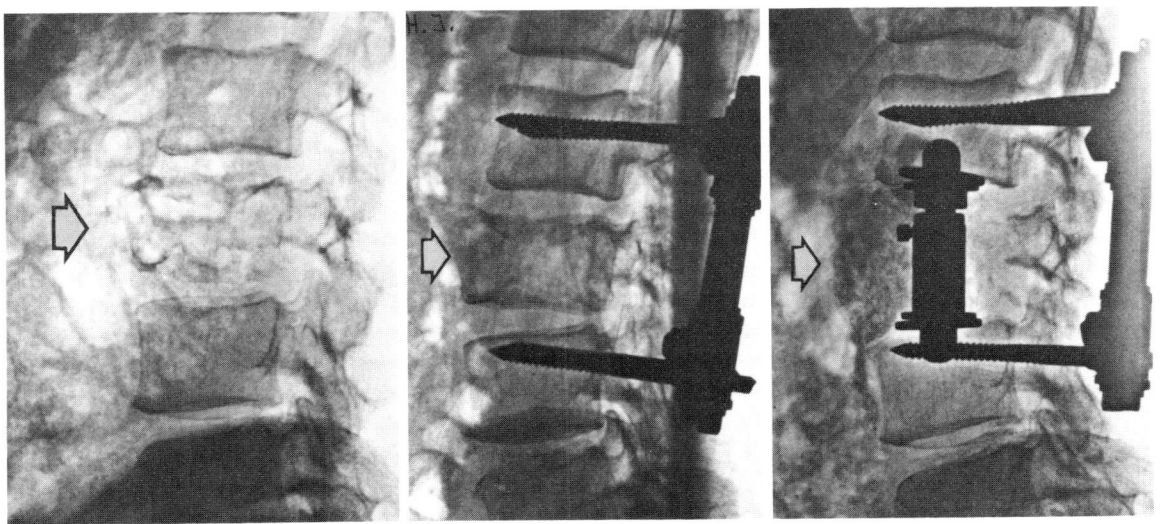

Fig. 93. Internal fixator used to bridge a vertebra infiltrated by malignant fibrositic histiocytoma. The vertebral body was then resected and a prosthesis used to replace it (patient H.J., male, 40 years old).

91

Where a primary vertebral tumor or solitary metastasis is present and resection of the body or vertebrectomy (excision of the entire vertebra) is planned, the fixator may be used. This makes the operation safer and followup treatment simpler and less unpleasant for the patient. Initially, the two adjacent vertebra are instrumented and this may need to be preceded by resection of the dorsal elements of the vertebra affected by the tumor including the pedicles. If there is reduction in the vertebral height, it can be restored by parallel distraction with the clamps firmly tightened, or it may be fixed in situ. The patient is then repositioned and the vertebral body resected from an anterior approach. The adjacent vertebral bodies are spread somewhat, and the vertebral replacement of ceramic, metal, cement or bone is anchored between the end plates. In this way, an anterior column capable of load bearing is restored, and the fixator stabilizes against rotation and translation forces.

The patient can be mobilized within a few days since pain should be abolished and the spine should be stable. Figure 93 shows such an example.

## 9.4 Degenerative and iatrogenic vertebral column instability

Painful instability of the lumbar spine due to degeneration of intervertebral discs is not uncommonly treated by posterolateral fusion, especially when more than one intervertebral disc is affected. If there is root compression due to narrowing of the intervertebral foramina, or protrusion of the discs, restoration of the original anatomical intervertebral height is desired using distraction. Here, parallel distraction of the affected segments can be precisely performed using the internal fixator without an undesired kyphosis. Simultaneous fusion of the transverse processes and arches is not impaired by the implant. Routine removal of the implant is recommended in these cases, since micromovements do occur between the vertebral bodies even where there is a stable posterolateral bony fusion, and the implant may fatigue or loosen in the long term.

After neurosurgical decompressive procedures in which the intervertebral joints may also be removed bilaterally, instability may develop postoperatively. This can be prevented with a fixator, which stabilizes the affected segment, and this should be combined with an intertransverse or a posterior interbody fusion across the disc space.

## 9.5 Spondylolistheses

If a spondylolisthesis progresses, or continues to be painful despite conservative treatment, fusion of the motion segment is indicated. The surgeon is confronted with the problem that a posterolateral fusion in an adolescent will not prevent the possibility of further angular deformity, because even a firm posterior fusion mass can be deformed by remodelling. On the other hand, interbody fusion often results in pseudarthrosis.

If the spondylolisthesis is greater than 50% or even a 100%, should the deformity be reduced, or an in-situ fusion performed? In order to cure pain, reduction is not necessary. Usually the pain stops as soon as solid fusion has occurred, and this is also usually true of pre-existing neurological symptoms. However, reduction improves the chance of a fusion occurring. Only reduction will correct the abnormal shape of the spine and posture, but there is always a danger of neurological injury. In view of these problems, it is not surprising that there are many differing views on the management of this problem in the literature [19, 36, 41, 51, 66, 72, 108, 132, 175, 180, 213, 222, 223].

The main aim of this section is to demonstrate the possibilities offered by the use of the internal fixator. If we assume that surgery is indicated at all, the aims of surgical treatment are in order of importance:
a) solid bony fusion between the unstable vertebra and sacrum,
b) preservation of mobility of the rest of the spine,
c) improvement in the position of the spine

a) *Solid bony fusion:* An anterior interbody fusion is more reliable biomechanically than a posterolateral fusion. Once consolidated, it will not fail in the long term, neither due to remodelling nor due to a fatigue fracture or trauma. However, in a spondylolisthesis an anterior interbody

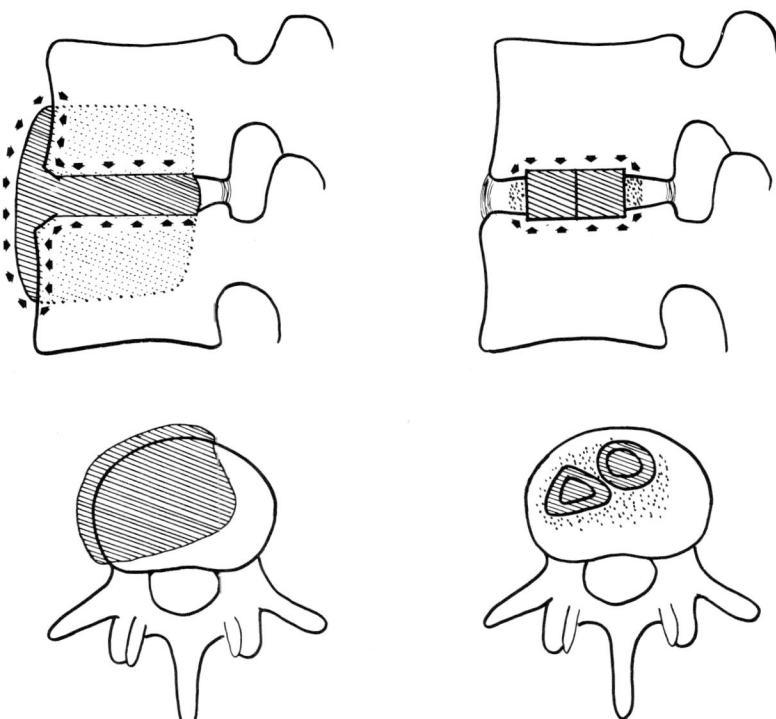

Fig. 94. Scheme of anterior fusion using bone paste compared with intercorporeal corticocancellous graft. There is a larger contact area, vascularization simultaneously from all sides, and a mechanically favorable position further away from the axis of rotation.

fusion is more difficult to obtain because of the greater displacement and poor mechanics, and because of the difficulty of external immobilization.

There are two methods of favorably influencing consolidation, firstly improving the technique of fusion, and secondly, ensuring complete mechanical rest during the healing phase with a stable implant. The internal fixator has proved to be a satisfactory implant applied from L 5 to S 1 as shown by the figures in this section. The patients can be mobilized at one week. The technique of interbody fusion which we have developed will be dealt with in more detail. Instead of a cortical bone block which is only slowly incorporated from the two end plates, we use autologous bone graft which has been finely ground into a paste as described in Section 8.3. The end plates are roughened up with a curette, but in addition, the anterior longitudinal ligament and the anterior anulus fibrosus are completely resected. The anterior edges of the vertebral bodies are nibbled away and the periosteum is stripped off from the anterior sur-

faces of L 5 and S 1. The bone graft is then used to fill the intervertebral space as well as covering the anterior walls of L 5 and S 1 as demonstrated in Figure 94. This has the advantage of enlarging the contact area between the bone graft and the vertebrae, and the surface area of the bone graft is increased many times. Vascularization of the bone graft takes place simultaneously over its entire surface from the bone and from the retroperitoneum. The shell-like connection which results between the two vertebrae is very stable mechanically due to its shape and its anterior position with a large lever arm from the center of rotation of the motion segment. 15 consecutive cases treated with this technique developed a stable callus-like bone graft anteriorly within 12 weeks without exception and a mature bony bridge developed within 9 months. This is demonstrated in Figures 95, 96, 99 and 100.

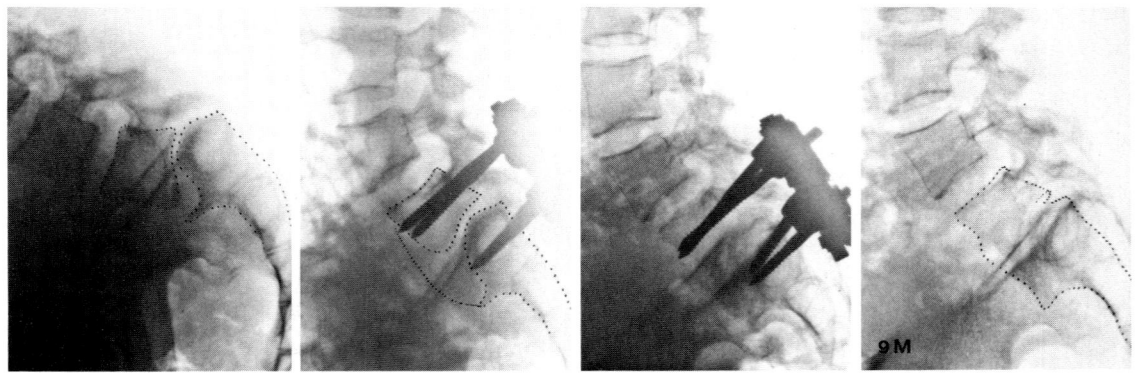

Fig. 95. Anterior release, anterior fusion with autologous bone paste, dorsal reduction and stabilization using the internal fixator. Rapid consolidation with removal of the fixator after eight months (patient, H.C., female, 17 years old).

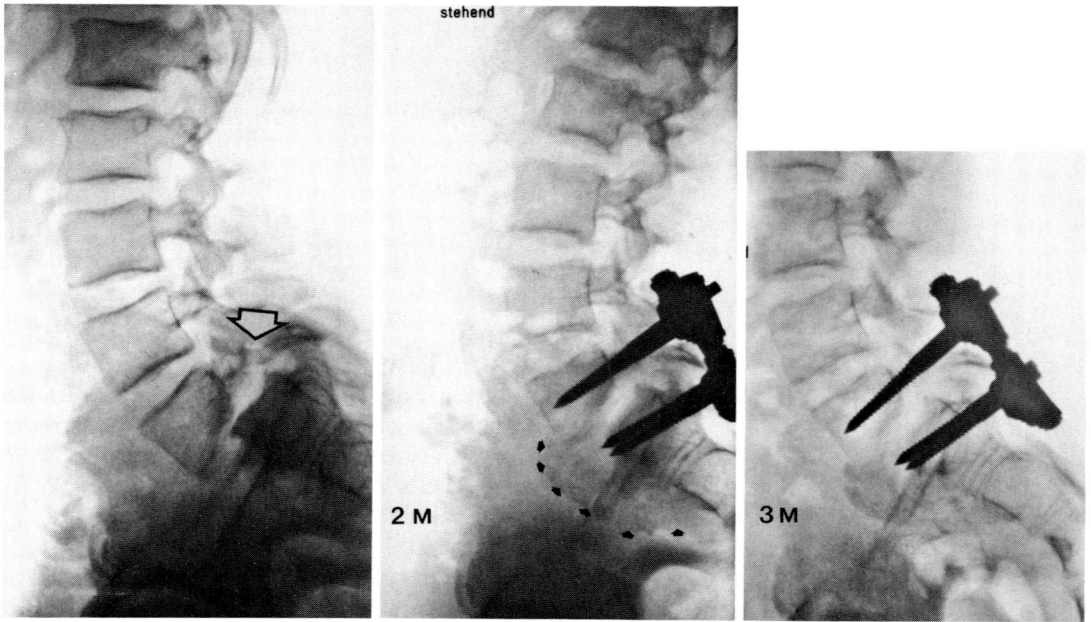

Fig. 96. Same procedure as in Figure 95. Large consolidating fusion mass anterior to S1 as early as two months. Patient mobilized postoperatively from the seventh day (patient, H.F., male, 15 years old).

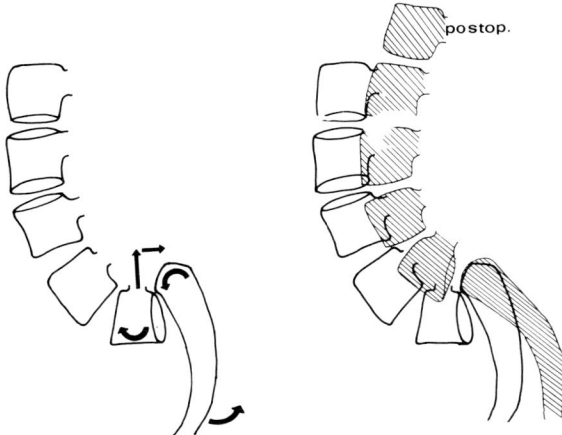

postop.

Fig. 97. Reduction of a spondyloptosis consists of complex movements in which the lordosis between L5 and S1 is restored. This is crucial for normal spinal function.

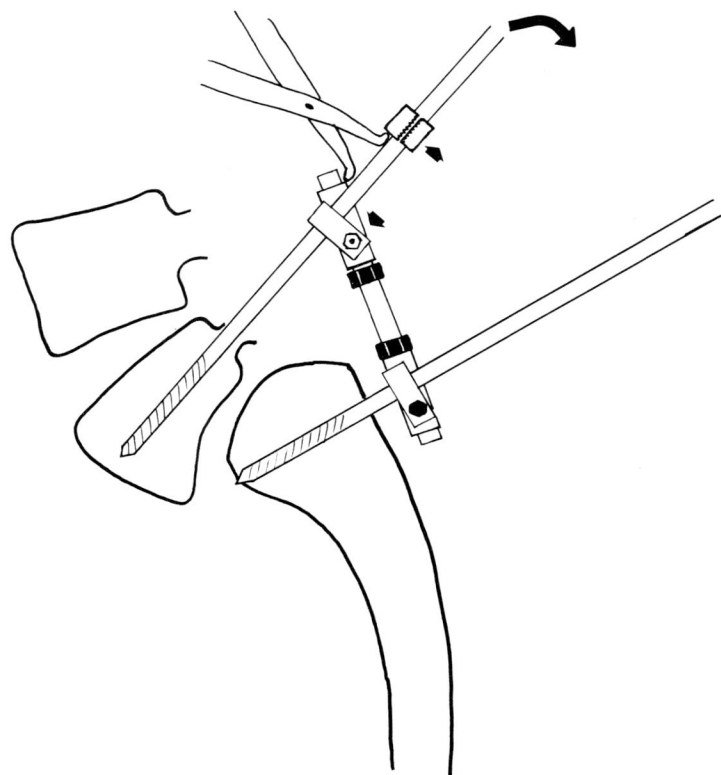

Fig. 98. Scheme of the technique of reduction. The fixator rod is tightened on the Schanz screw in S1 in such a way that it stands off some distance posterior to L5. L5 is then drawn posteriorly towards the fixator rod using the spreaders and manual lordosis is performed simultaneously. The distraction nut opposed to the clamp element ensures simultaneous distraction during lordosis.

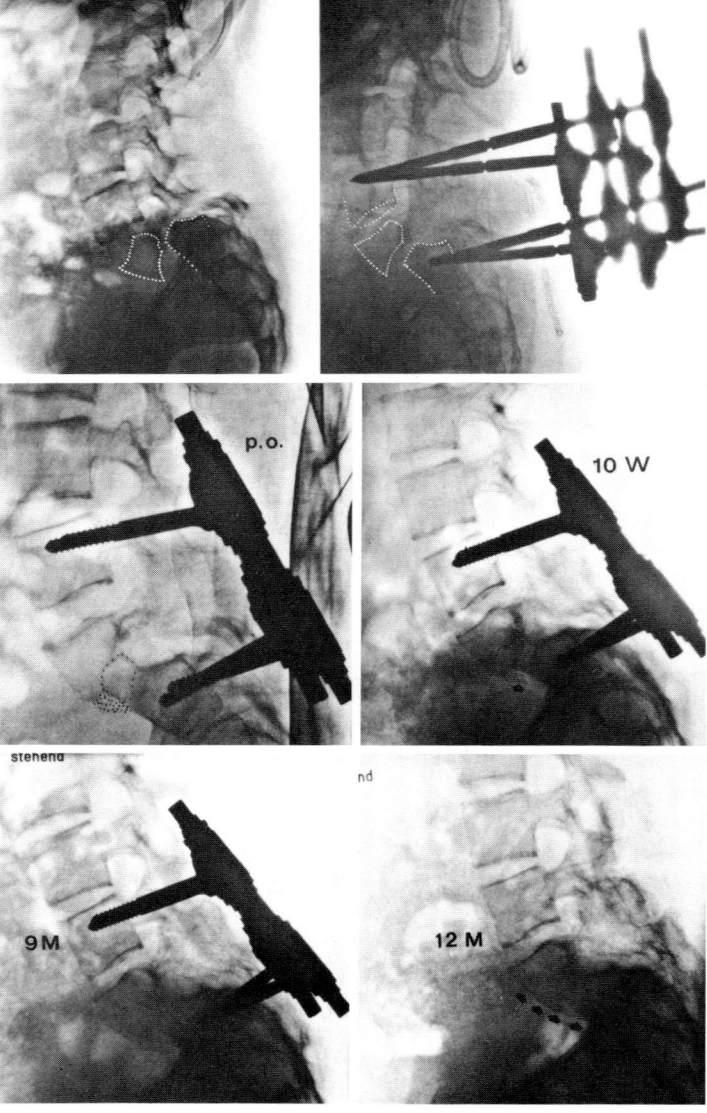

Fig. 99. Two-stage procedure in spondyloptosis. Initial slow reduction using the external fixator with screws in L4 and S1 over a period of 14 days with neurological monitoring. In the second procedure, anterior fusion and dorsal reduction and stabilization using the internal fixator are performed. Rapid ossification (patient A.D., female, 12 years old).

b) *Preservation of the mobility of the rest of the lumbar spine:* In contrast to scoliosis, the deformity in spondylolisthesis is restricted to one segment. The rest of the spine only shows compensatory alterations in position, but has a relatively normal function. As in fracture treatment, arthrodesis should be restricted to the pathological level. This idea is not new, but was overshadowed by the widespread use of Harrington instrumentation. As early as 1975, SCHÖLLNER [175] presented his one level fixation

reduction using sacral plates and transpedicular screws in the 5th lumbar vertebra. This was one of the very early applications of pedicle screws outside of fracture treatment. In France, LOUIS [108] always advocated fixation of only the lumbosacral junction.

Harrington distraction systems are usually applied to L3 or even as high as L2 and L1, but this is undesirable functionally and is not necessary. Well proven procedures have been described which do not affect the remainder of the lumbar

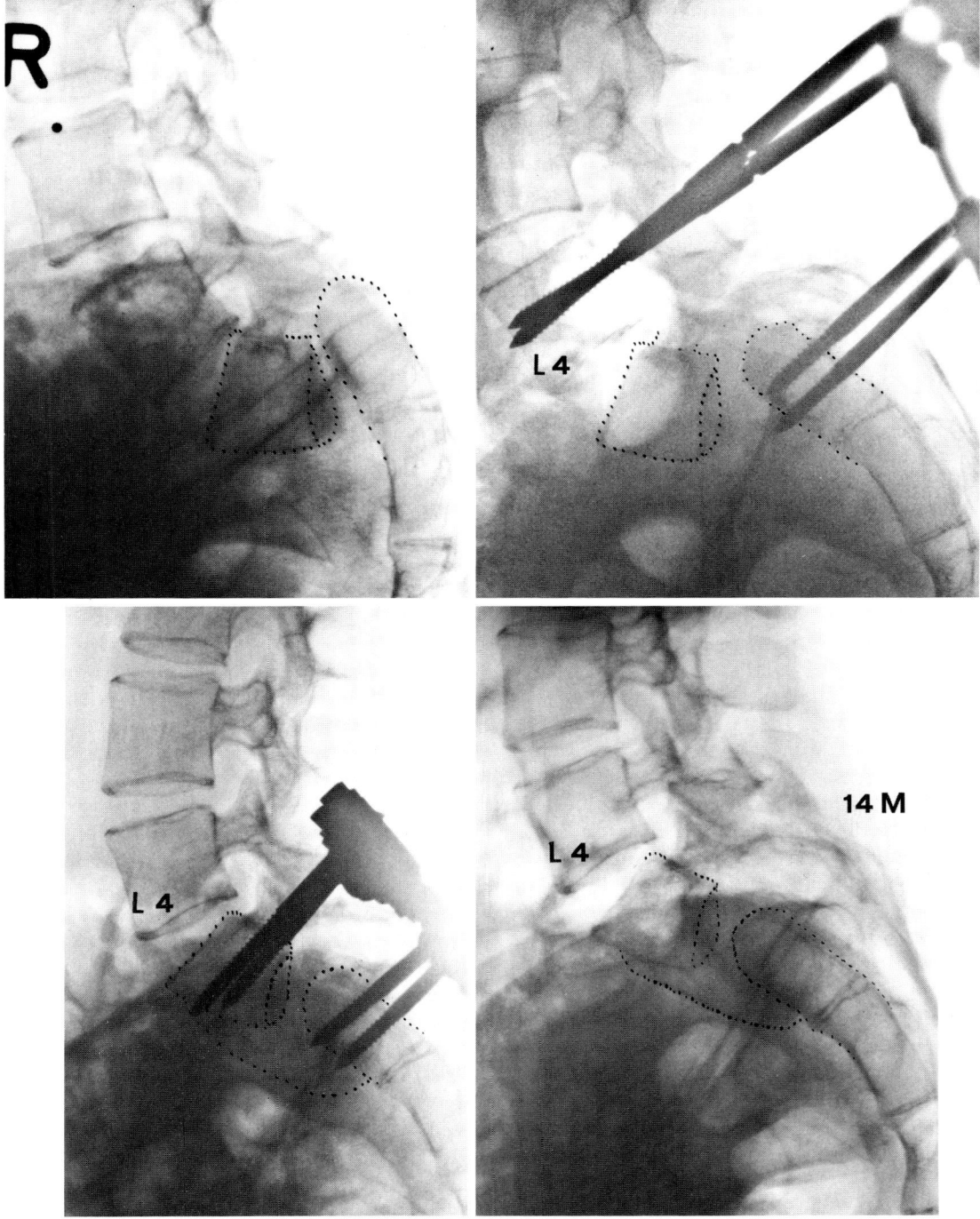

Fig. 100. Same procedure as in Fig. 99. In the second procedure when the internal fixator is being applied, the Schanz screws are switched to L5. Thus a monosegmental L5/S1 fusion results (patient S.U., female, 18 years old).

spine, and these include anterior instrumentation [108], posterior instrumentation [145] and combined instrumentation [66, 108]. Instrumentation using the internal fixator can be compared with these methods.

Occasionally, it is necessary to instrument the fourth lumbar vertebra because L5 cannot be reached. This happens only in complete spondyloptosis.

c) *Improvement in spine shape:* The anatomy of the spine is impaired in severe spondylolisthesis by anterior displacement of the trunk and its center of gravity, with a compensatory hyperlordosis extending high into the thoracic spine. The sacrum becomes more vertical, the deformity itself being *kyphotic.*

Hence the Harrington instrumentation is unsuitable for biomechanical reasons, quite apart from the length of the implant. Additional devices attached to the rod pulling L5 dorsally are not satisfactory biomechanically either [180]. The distraction force cannot eliminate the vertical position of the sacrum nor the anterior displacement of the more proximal spine, even if it is possible to reduce at least partially the lower lumbar vertebral body which has slid forward in front of the sacrum in a spondyloptosis.

The position of the spine would be improved by correction of the kyphosis of the sliding vertebra in relation to the sacrum. This is more important than elimination of the displacement in the a. p. direction.

Figure 97 shows the components necessary for complete reduction of a spondyloptosis. One can either say that the sacrum must be rotated under L5 or L5 must be rotated in relation to the sacrum. The Schanz screws of the fixator are very suitable for such tilting movement, so that the fixator may be used for reduction as well as for stabilization of the fusion in spondylolisthesis.

The details of the procedure in cases where the lumbosacral intervertebral discs can be reached anteriorly (i. e. with about 80% displacement or less) are as follows. Autologous bone paste is obtained from the posterior aspect of the ilium as described in Section 8.3. The patient is then placed in a supine position, and through a transperitoneal approach an «anterior release» is performed. This involves resection of the anterior longitudinal ligament as well as the anterior and lateral parts of the anulus fibrosus and the intervertebral disc itself. Quite often the lower edge of L5 needs to be chiseled off in order to gain access. The end plates are roughened up and the periosteum anterior to L5 and S1 is excised. The autologous bone graft is inserted as described previously. The graft does not need to be attached, and the parietal peritoneum is closed with continuous suturing. Intra-abdominal pressure after closure of the abdominal wall holds the graft in place. The advantage of this is that changes in position of the vertebrae can be carried out without danger of displacing a cortical graft from its bed, which would compromise the fusion. The bone paste follows any change of position due to the vacuum effect. Thus reduction can be carried out through a posterior approach, and this is facilitated by the anterior release.

The third part of the operation is carried out under the same anesthetic, although it is conceivable that it could be performed a few days later. A conventional midline dorsal approach is made with the patient prone. Experience shows that the transpedicular screws should be placed more cranial than usual in L5, lateral to the L4/5 intervertebral joints instead of below them. Trial placement with a thin Kirschner wire and image intensifier control is very important here. Instrumentation of the sacrum and the problems of positioning are dealt with in Section 8.1.

Figure 98 shows a possible way of applying the necessary reduction forces. After applying the short threaded rods, these are fixed with the lateral nuts on the lower Schanz screws in such a way that the rods are elevated proximally about 2 cms from the bone. The distraction nuts on the threaded rods are approximated to the clamp elements, so that distraction arises while lordosing. An additional free clamp element is now fixed on the cranial Schanz screw. An arthrodesis spreader is placed between this and the rod and is used to press the proximal end of the threaded rod towards the bone. By this, L5 is pulled posteriorly. At the same time, a lordosis is applied to the Schanz screws in L5 and hence to the vertebra itself. The upper clamp is then tightened using the lateral nut. One side is done at a time, and this can be repeated alternately several times as necessary. Simultaneously, scoliosis can be eliminated by differential distraction.

98

In a spondylolisthesis greater than 80–100% where the lumbosacral intervertebral disc cannot be appproached from anteriorly, the procedure needs modification. In adults, this is best restricted to correction of L4 by lordotic L4/S1 instrumentation and a posterolateral fusion. In adolescents, reduction can be achieved in the following way. At a preliminary operation, the Schanz screws are inserted through the skin into S1 and L4. L5 is almost vertical and is not accessible. The Schanz screws are now connected outside the body with an external fixator frame or with two internal fixator rods on each side. Daily adjustment of the fixator allows slow and gentle reduction of the deformity using distraction and lordosis, over a period of about two weeks, and the patient can be monitored neurologically throughout. When the 5th lumbar vertebral body is sufficiently reduced, an anterior interbody fusion is carried out as a second procedure, and further reduction is performed dorsally, now using an internal fixator instrumentation, first on one side and then on the other. Figure 99 shows an example. In certain circumstances, the Schanz screws may be removed from L4 and placed in L5, once L5 becomes more accessible (Fig. 100).

Lumbosacral instrumentations in spondylolisthesis and particularly in spondyloptosis are by far the most difficult procedures. They require the greatest experience clinically and also experience with the implant.

## 9.6 Lumbosacral malformations

Earlier attempts to correct lumbosacral malformations with wedged lumbar vertebral bodies using a short Harrington distraction rod to the sacrum on the concave side, and a compression device on the convex side have not been successful at our institution. It was not possible to render the end plate horizontal, probably because these implants act eccentrically on the dorsal elements. The instrumentation was not adequate to correct the deformity in three dimensions. Provided that no bony malunion is present, three dimensional correction of spinal deformity can be attained using the internal fixator, because of the forces which can be applied in almost any direction. Figure 101 shows a case where a 25° sagittal deformity of L5 relative to L6 was corrected using the internal fixator. This was performed dorsally without anterior release, and was held by a posterolateral fusion. In this case, previous X-rays had shown a pre-existing lumbosacral malformation present before the onset of a progressive scoliosis. This case is only an example to show one of the applications

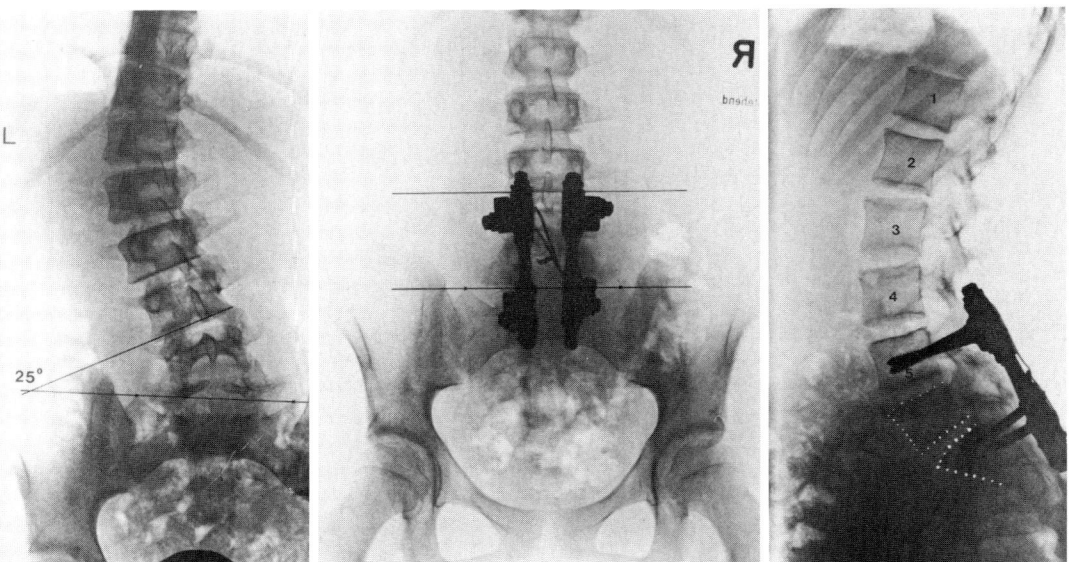

Fig. 101. Example of a disorder of the lumbosacral junction with 25° lateral tilting of L5 and lateral deviation of the trunk. Correction of the deformity with the internal fixator, see text (patient N. V., female, 14 years old).

of the internal fixator as an instrument for reducing deformity, but it should not tempt us to treat the more frequent primary lumboscolioses with this type of fixation.

### 9.7 Salvage procedures

In spinal surgery, there are unusual individual cases which are not included in the usual indications for surgery using standard procedures, but where surgery needs to be adapted to the in-dividual case. In some cases, the properties of the internal fixator can be exploited to solve these problems. Three cases are described in detail as examples.

a) The 45-year-old, female patient shown in Figure 102 sustained a fracture of the 10th thoracic vertebra with complete paraplegia. Many years later, a grotesque unstable deformity developed at the thoracolumbar junction two vertebrae below the original injury, with a kyphosis of 35 and a lateral deformity of 45 (a

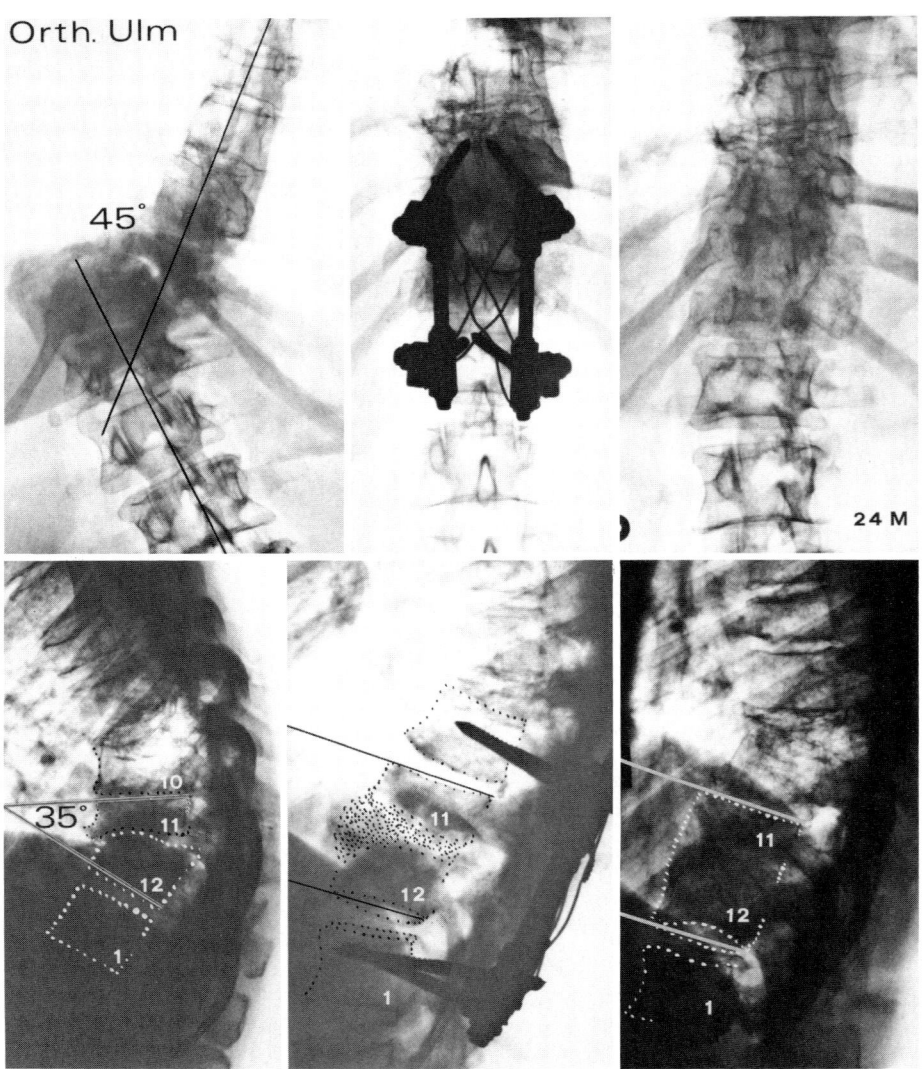

Fig. 102. Charcot spine two levels below a vertebral fracture associated with paraplegia. Correction of the deformity using the internal fixator with preservation of mobility of the entire lumbar spine. Interbody fusion through the dorsal approach. The torsion is not corrected (patient S.G., female, 45 years old). With kind permission of Prof. PUHL, Ulm.

Charcot spine). The deformity was so severe that the patient was hardly able to sit normally. The aim of treatment was to eliminate the deformity while maintaining stability of the correction until consolidation of the interbody fusion had occurred, and yet to preserve full mobility of the lumbar spine. It was relatively simple to instrument the spine using the internal fixator, and for the last two years the patient has been able to sit normally.

b) The patient shown in Figure 103 was a 74-year-old man who had a «failed back surgery syndrome» after multiple disc hernia operations, laminectomies and attempted fusions. Uncontrollable lumbar pain associated with onset of abnormal neurology were the indications for surgery. After extensive canal and root decompression, the lumbar spine was stabilized using a distracting fixator rod on the concave side and a compressing fixator rod on the convex side. The patients back pain improved markedly, although he did not become pain free. He subsequently died from another cause two years later.

c) Figure 104 shows radiographs of a 63-year-old patient with a rapidly progressive paraparesis which occurred 10 days after a staphylococcal septicemia combined with a pleural abscess, which arose due to osteomyelitis of the metatarsum. A T9–11 laminectomy was carried out elsewhere. The osteolysis seen in T9 increased despite antibiotic therapy, and a further focus of infection became visible at T10–11. The patient was transferred for resection of the infected area. Excision of the infected focus by anterior approach with cancellous bone grafting led as expected to consolidation of the bone graft within a few months and fusion. However, due to the previous laminectomy there was a danger of instability in association with the anterior resection and there was a fear that it would lead to neurological deterioration.

Initially, a long internal fixator was used to stabilize the spine and subsequently extensive focal resection (hatched area seen in Fig.104) and cancellous bone grafting was carried out via a thoractomy. Healing and bony consolidation were uneventful and the implant was removed two years later.

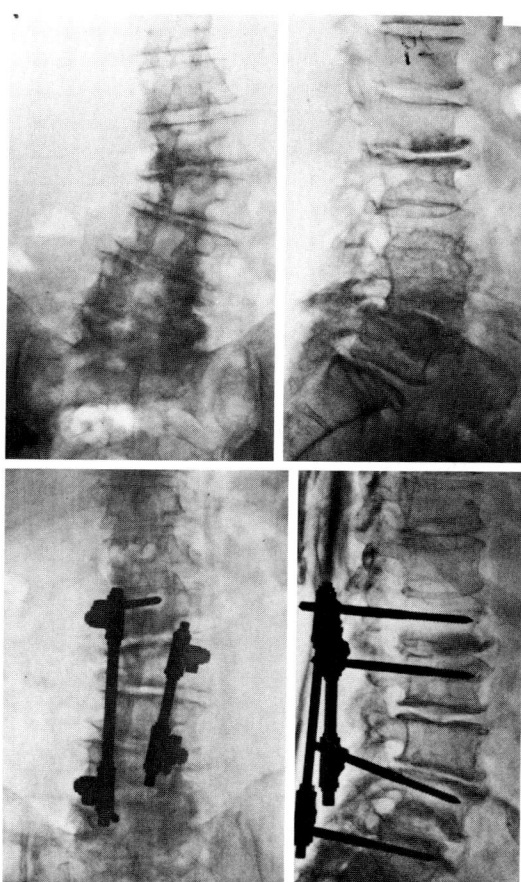

Fig.103. «Failed back surgery syndrome» after multiple operations, see text (patient W.H., male, 74 years old).

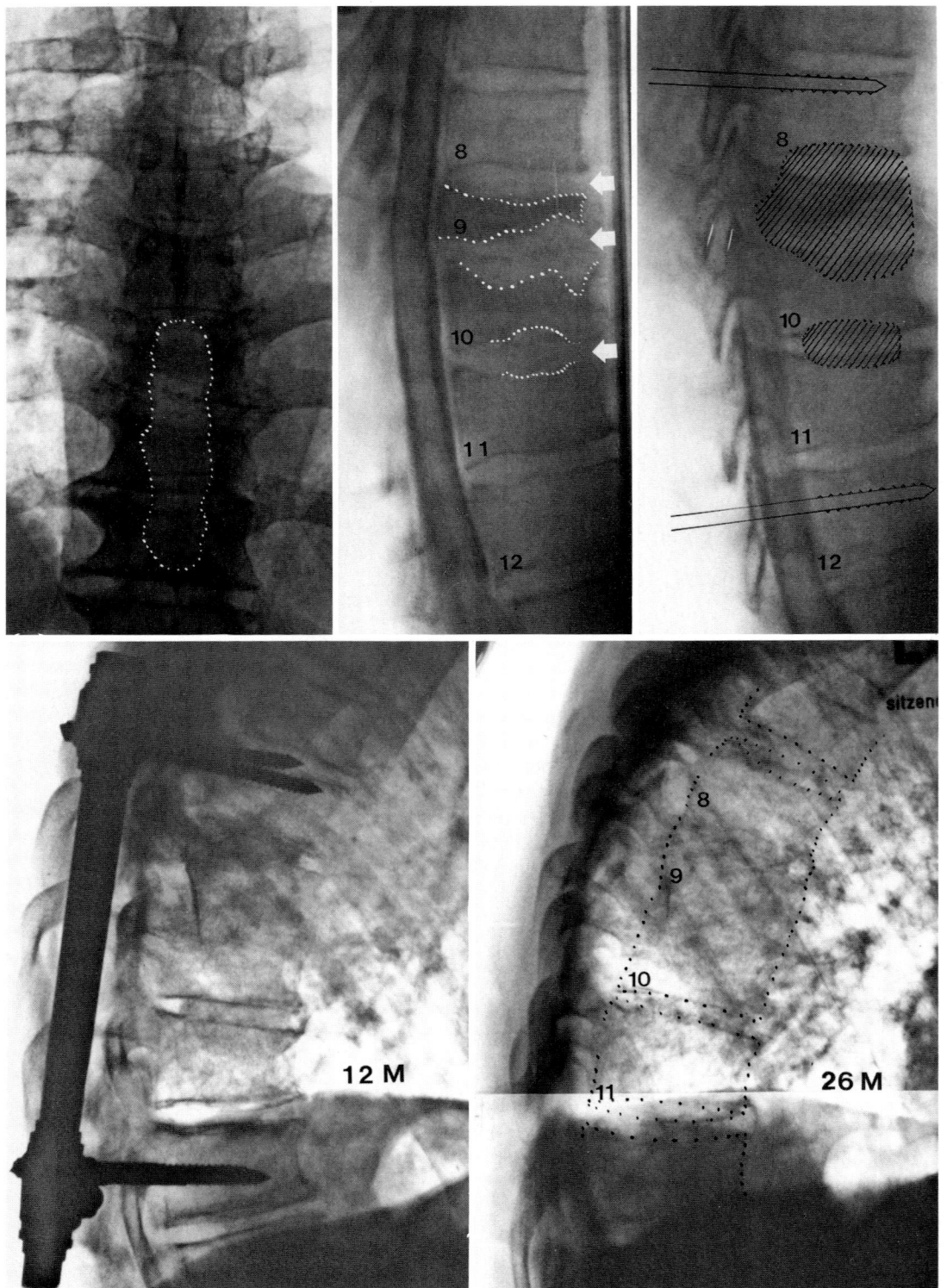

Fig. 104. Pre-existing T9-11 laminectomy. Infection of T9, with a new focus of infection in T10/11 disc space. Anterior resection of T9 by thoracotomy and excision of infected material at the T10/11 space, subsequent to prior stabilization using an internal fixator. The infection healed, the spine consolidated, and the implant was removed two years later (patient C.M., male, 63 years old).

## 10. Results

The above observations are based on the following clinical experience:

### 10.1 Patients and results of follow-up investigations

From December 1982 to October 1986, 183 patients were treated with instrumentation using the internal fixator at the Orthopedics Division, University of Basle. They have been regularly followed up. The shortest period of observation is six months and the longest 52 months. In 80 cases, the duration of observation exceeds two years. As far as possible we have contacted patients abroad and have received written reports, so that the follow-up is complete. Indications for surgery are as follows:

| | |
|---|---:|
| Fractures | 111 |
| Posttraumatic deformities and instabilities | 20 |
| Tumors and metastases | 11 |
| Degenerative and iatrogenic spinal instabilities | 16 |
| Spondylolistheses | 16 |
| Salvage procedures | 4 |
| Other indications (malformations, scolioses) | 5 |
| | 183 |

Ten surgeons were involved, i.e. the more experienced members of the hospital staff covering the emergency service were responsible operatively, demonstrating that the procedure can be learned by any spinal surgeon.

### 10.1.1 Fractures

Of the 111 patients in this group, 84 were men and 27 were women. The average age was 34, the minimum age was 15 years and the maximum 76 years. Of the 111 patients, 10 had sustained a second major fracture requiring treatment in the region of the thoracic or lumbar spine.

In three of them, the fractures were far apart, and two separate internal fixators were used, namely for T7 and L3, for T12 and L3, and for L1 and L4. In six patients two adjacent vertebrae were affected so that one additional segment was included in the fixation. In one case, the second fracture was treated above the internal fixator with a monosegmental Harrington compression instrumentation (Fig. 78). The levels of the 121 instumented fractures were as follows.

| | |
|---|---:|
| T4: | 1 |
| T5: | 1 |
| T6: | 1 |
| T7: | 2 |
| T8: | 1 |
| T9: | 3 |
| T10: | 1 |
| T11: | 6 |
| T12: | 27 |
| L1: | 46 |
| L2: | 16 |
| L3: | 10 |
| L4: | 5 |
| L5: | 1 |
| | 121 |

The average kyphotic angle of the fractured vertebra was 20.4°. It should be noted that most patients were radiographed in a position where the fractures were partially reduced. Postoperatively, the average kyphotic angle was 5.1°. In one case, there was no consolidation of the fracture, and a further anterior procedure was necessary six months later, as mentioned below under Complications. In all the other cases, the fracture consolidated. It was gratifying that there was little compression of the fractured vertebrae during consolidation. At final followup in each

103

case, there was an average loss of correction within the vertebral body of only 1° (minimum 0° maximum 15°). However, loss of height of the intervertebral disc was frequently seen after removal of the implant at the level of the injury. This occurred in the absence of an anterior bony bridge. This narrowing of the intervertebral disc led to kyphosis of 2°–4°: an example is shown in Figure 105. The implant has been removed in 70 patients.

Anteroposterior subluxations can be reduced well using the fixator. Residual anterior or posterior displacement of 3 mm or more was accepted intraoperatively in only a few patients in whom a complete division of the canal contents was found. All the remaining displacements were reduced to less than 3 mm.

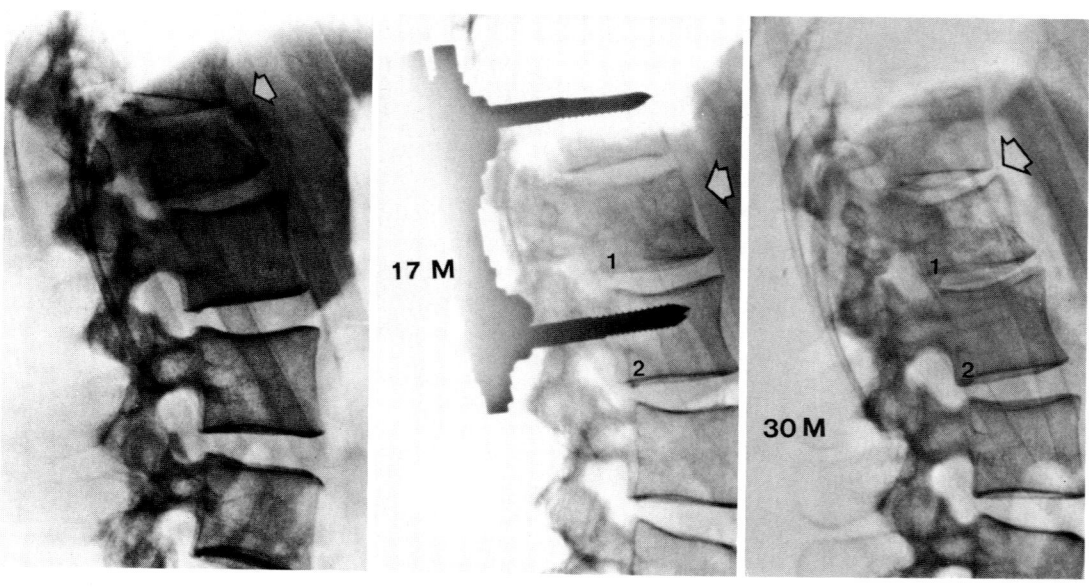

Fig. 105. An average of only 1 degree of further kyphosis occurred in the vertebral bodies filled with cancellous bone. However, reduction in height at the adjacent intervertebral space was almost always present with a kyphosis of less than 5°, unless the disc space is bridged by bone (patient B.D., female, 36 years old).

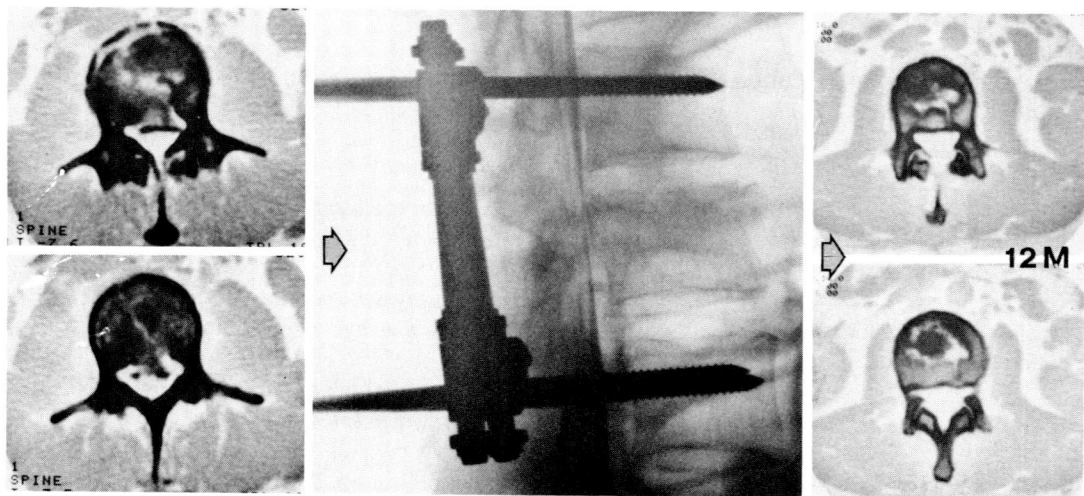

Fig. 106. Reduction of the posterior wall fragment using the internal fixator instrumentation without opening the vertebral canal (patient C.N., female, 23 years old). CT scan on the right after implant removal.

We do not have a large enough number of pre- and postoperative computerized tomograms to be statistically significant. Figures 79 and 106 show individual examples.

Most impressive are the functional results, which are difficult to express numerically and are best shown on video. Within three to four months of injury, paraplegic patients were able to climb back into their wheelchair after a fall to the ground. This is only possible with a very mobile lumbar spine. The physiotherapists and the rehabilitation specialists agree that the functional results are generally as good as in conservative treatment. In contrast, implants which cross many segments provide less good results.

The neurological status of the patients with spine fractures should also be discussed. Neurological recovery after transverse lesions is always cited as justification for certain surgical techniques. However, it is clear that recovery depends on the extent of the primary injury, together with the pathophysiological processes which have resulted in the spinal cord. The completeness and the timing of decompression may influence recovery, but the techniques by which it has been reached are less important. With so many variables, the individual surgeon is hardly able to compare different regimes statistically. The presentation of the neurological status of the patients in this work purely documents the fact that, by using the internal fixator, the paraplegic patient has equally good chances of recovery compared with other methods.

Ninety of the patients with fractures had neurological impairment and were treated postoperatively in the Swiss Paraplegia Center in Basle. Rehabilitation has been completed in all patients. According to the Frankel classification, they had the following distribution.

Frankel A: 23 patients
Frankel B: 9 patients
Frankel C: 29 patients
Frankel D: 29 patients

After rehabilitation (average 158 days), the following patients had improved by at least one Frankel stage:

from A: 5 out of 23 patients (22%)
from B: 4 out of 9 patients (44%)
from C: 23 out of 29 patients (78%)

_____

31 out of 61 patients (51%)

The initial Frankel staging was carried out according to very strict criteria, and in stage A there was no sacral sparing. However, many of these patients had been admitted to hospital and operated on within a few hours of injury before the bulbocavernosus reflex had returned, and the 5 patients who improved may have had B lesions and still been in spinal shock.

In group D, most patients had neurological improvement. However with careful neurological examination small residual defects were frequently found. Incidentally the Frankel classification is not very suitable for precise analyses and in the future, separate records of motor and sensory activity would be helpful.

The patients in Frankel groups A–C were mobilized on average 22 days after the injury in a wheelchair (minimum 5 days, maximum 73 days). Those in groups D and E could walk or stand after an average of 13 days (minimum 1 day, maximum 52 days). The longer duration in both groups can be explained by the high proportion of polytraumatized patients and bilateral fractures of the lower limbs.

At follow-up, four patients had commited suicide six months to two years after the injury. These are not listed among the complications. In all these patients also the vertebral fracture had been caused by an attempted suicide.

## 10.1.2 Posttraumatic deformities and instabilities

There were 20 patients in this group, of whom 10 were men and 10 were women. The average age was 28 with a minimum of 17 and a maximum of 54 years. The original trauma had occurred three to 12 months previously. 11 patients had undergone prior conservative treatment, seven patients had failed posterior surgery (4 Harrington, 1 Luque, 1 locking hook spinal rod, 1 facet screw fixation). Two patients had undergone anterior fusion. The fracture levels involved were as follows;

T 5: 2
T 12: 2
L 1: 11
L 2: 2
L 3: 1
L 4: 1
L 5: 1

In these cases, surgery was indicated for back pain due to deformity or non-union. In all these patients, posterolateral fusion was carried out simultaneously, and in every case fusion has occurred. Half the patients have already had the metal work removed. Three patients had an anterior spinal osteotomy at the same time, and all of these have likewise healed. One female patient (T5) continued to have pain and one other patient had pain in the transitional region between the sensitive and non-sensitive area. The remainder are free of symptoms.

### 10.1.3 Tumors and metastases

This group consists of nine men and two women with an average age of 55 years (minimum 36, maximum 74 years). One patient is alive without recurrence 30 months after resection of a solitary plasmacytoma from L3. The other patients all died from their tumors two to 11 months postoperatively. These cases comprise one multiple myeloma, one undifferentiated carcinoma, two hypernephroma metastases, two breast cancer metastases, two bronchus carcinoma metastases and two adenocarcinoma metastases.

One patient was and remained paraplegic. The remaining patients only displayed incipient neurological symptoms, and there was good recovery postoperatively. Two patients with a survival time of two months could not be mobilized, but had less pain. The other patients were able to ambulate for a considerable period of time and were discharged home for months in most cases.

### 10.1.4 Degenerative and iatrogenic spinal instabilities

Seven men and nine women in this group had an average age of 57 years (minimum 28, maximum 82 years). Instrumentation with the internal fixator stabilized nine especially wide laminectomies with degenerative stenoses as well as degenerative spondylolistheses. Seven patients had chronic lumbar pain syndrome due to spondyloarthrosis and disc problems. Five of them had already had disc surgery, in some cases at several levels. The lower lumbar spine was involved in all cases. In four cases, the fixation was restricted to one motion segment only, 11 cases were instrumented over two segments as is usually the case, and one was over three segments. In nine cases, the distal screws were placed in the sacrum, in five cases in L5 and in two cases in L4. Lateral fusions were performed in all cases. All the patients were mobilized within a week, and their recovery was as for the fracture patients.

### 10.1.5 Spondylolistheses

This group consists of two male and 14 female patients with an average age of 22 (minimum 12, maximum 48).

The anterior displacement of L5 on S1 averaged 72% (minimum 45%, maximum 110%). Reduction was carried out leaving an average residual displacement of 31% (minimum 0%, maximum 50%).

The average correction of the kyphosis of L5 in relation to the sacrum was 32° (minimum 10°, maximum 65°). This was referred to in Section 9.5 because of its extreme importance regarding spinal posture. The stability of the internal fixator and the technique of fusion using autologous bone paste resulted in a firm fusion within 9 months in 13 of 14 cases of anterior fusion and two cases of posterolateral fusion. Implants have been removed from 12 patients. The average time of follow-up is 22 months (6–52 months), and to date no significant loss in the correction has been seen. All patients are completely painfree (pain being the main indication for surgery).

### 10.1.6. Salvage procedures

Case reports for these three patients were presented in Section 9.7. The fourth patient, a 20 year old man, with a high meningomyelocele, paralytic scoliosis and several previous operations, underwent combined anterior and posterior spinal osteotomy at L3 using the fixator in an atypical lateral position because of the huge CSF cavity. Wound healing and consolidation of the osteotomy occurred without complication.

### 10.1.7 Miscellaneous

Apart from the lumbosacral malformation described in Section 9.6, this group of five female patients included four adolescents with a short scoliosis at the thoracolumbar junction. In these cases a pedicular screw was used at the apex of the scoliosis, applying a derotational force as suggested by HEFTI [73a]. The patients were mobilized immediately without using a corset due to the stability of the instrumentation. As the followup period is only two years (20–34 months) and the patients are still growing, this group cannot be analysed comprehensively.

## 10.2 Complications

Among 183 consecutive patients followed for 6–52 months, the following complications were observed:

a) *One death secondary to pulmonary embolism on the 17th day:*

A 43-year-old man with multiple trauma including a T12/L1 fracture dislocation, multiple rib fractures and pneumothorax, a scapular fracture and complete paraplegia, was referred from another hospital four weeks after the injury, with decubitus ulcers on the heels and sacrum, as well as hepatitis B.

Due to his poor pulmonary function, the aim of treatment was to mobilize him and allow him to sit as soon as possible.

The dislocation was reduced using the internal fixator. The contents of the vertebral canal were seen to be completely divided at the time of surgery. The fixator was applied in the compression mode without restoration of vertebral height. Prophylactic anticoagulation was carried out with 5000 units of heparin three times daily without warfarin because of his hepatitis. On the 17th day postoperatively, he suffered a fatal pulmonary embolism.

At autopsy, the operation side was unremarkable. The spinal specimen with the fixator was tested using the material testing machine as described in Section 7.3. Subsequently, the specimen was dissected, and confirmed that the screws were in the correct position with a firm fit (Figs. 54, 55, 56).

b) *Three re-instrumentations using the same implant:*

In two patients, a satisfactory reduction was not attained initially. This was because distraction had been carried out initially, instead of eliminating the kyphosis and the subluxation first. One of the two cases was described in the section on surgical technique (8.1) as an example of the importance of the correct sequence of reduction; i.e. correction of the kyphosis first, followed by distraction. Adequate reduction was also achieved in the second case at reoperation with the correct technique. A transpedicular bone graft was performed, as shown in Figure 107.

In one case, a fracture of the Schanz screws required reoperation: In this 19 year old man, a fracture of the two upper screws occurred four months postoperatively with collapse of the vertebra. At reoperation, the kyphosis was again corrected with two new Schanz screws. The correction was carried out at the level of the intervertebral space as of course the height of the fractured vertebra could not be restored so long after the injury. Posterolateral fusion was performed and the fixator was removed one year later. 18 months after injury, the correction has been maintained (Fig. 108).

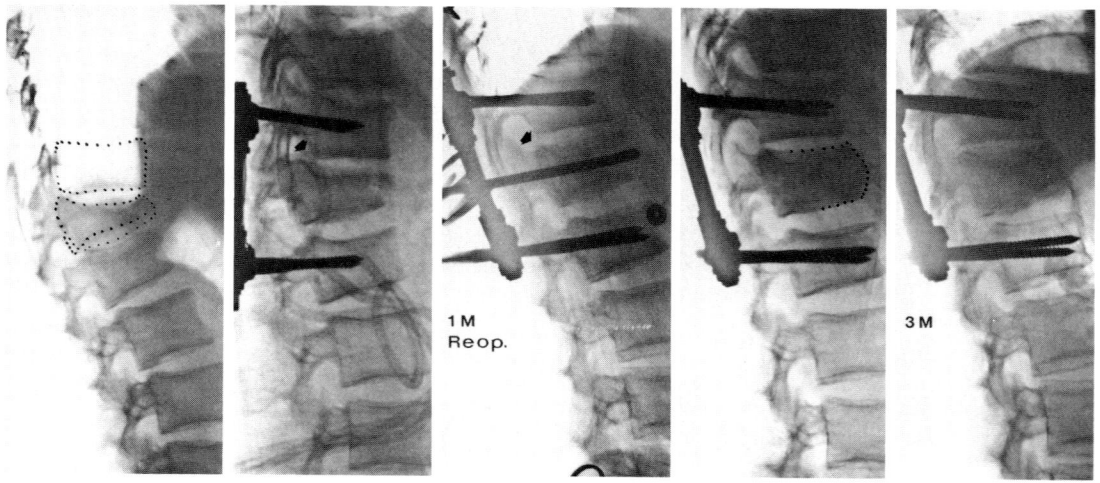

Fig. 107. Reduction was not successful at the initial operation, because distraction was carried out before correction of the kyphosis, with the result that the kyphosis is not correctable (cf. Section 8.1). At a second operation, the correct sequence of correction of the kyphosis followed by distraction as well as the obligatory cancellous bone grafting was performed (patient K.P., male, 17 years old).

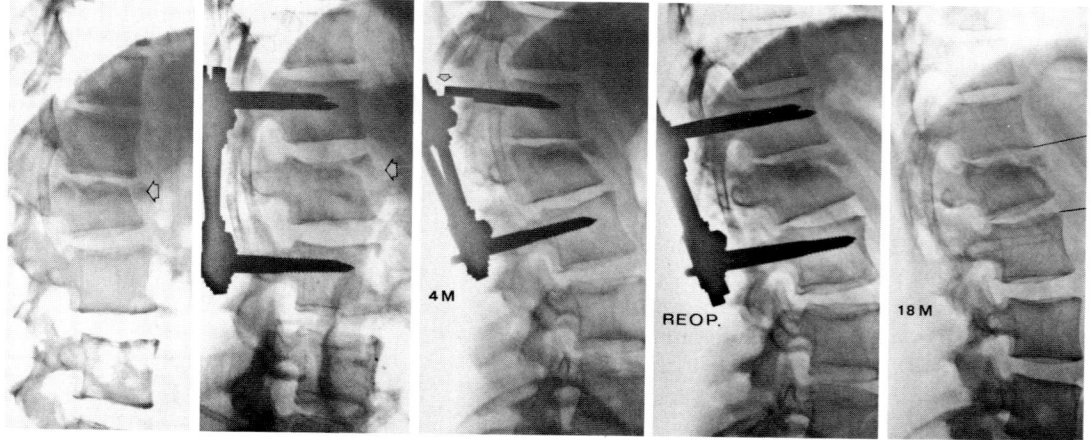

Fig. 108. The only reinstrumentation carried out for fracture of the Schanz screws four months postoperatively. On the right, result after 18 months (patient R.D., male, 19 years old).

c) *Switching to another implant:*

In an 18 year old patient with an L1 fracture, the fracture did not consolidate. The upper screws loosened with formation of a large cavity in the vertebral body of T12 six months later, so that anterior cancellous bone grafting and plate osteosynthesis was performed. The fixator was removed at the same time. This was the only case where another implant had to be used.

d) *Correction of the length of screw:*

In one case, one of the screws was placed too far anteriorly, beyond the anterior wall of the vertebra, due to poor visibility on the image intensifier (Fig. 109). The patient was asymptomatic, but nevertheless the screw was withdrawn using a stab incision. This is possible using the screw removing forceps from the instrument set without loosening the nut and clamp. The postoperative course was otherwise unremarkable and the fracture has since healed.

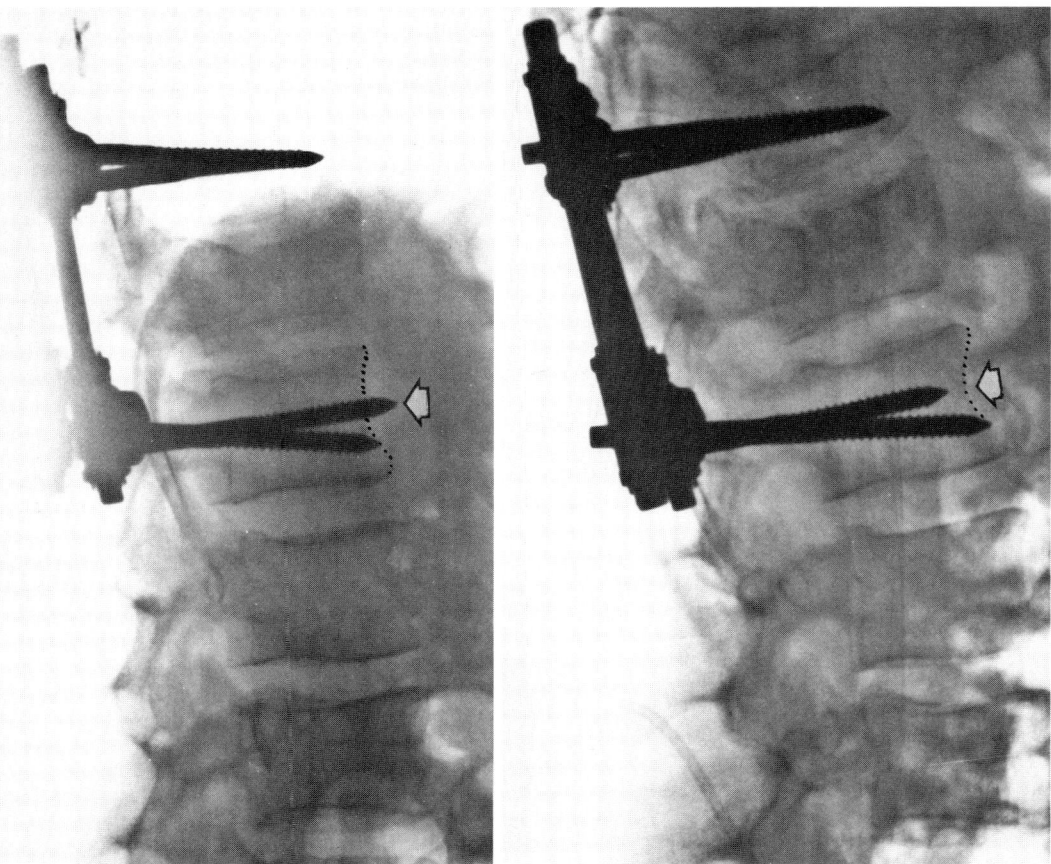

Fig. 109. For the sake of safety, the Schanz screw which is projecting anteriorly is withdrawn, cf. text (patient F. P., male, 30 years old).

### e) Two premature implant removals:

In two patients, the fixator was removed early on due to infection (one fracture, one degenerative instability). In the patient with the fracture, an anterior corrective bone graft was performed subsequently for correction of kyphosis, and the other patient was treated conservatively. In both cases, the infection healed without osteomyelitis.

Prophylactic administration of antibiotics during induction of anesthesia is worth considering. Vertebral fractures are frequently associated with extensive soft tissue trauma, and the implant lies in a contused area.

### f) Loss of correction:

In three patients, a secondary kyphosis of 10°–15° was observed within the first six weeks.

In two cases, this was probably caused by sinking of the Schanz screws into the cancellous bone of the vertebral body. In one case, a lateral malpositioning of the screw was shown.

In the 29 year old patient whose radiographs are shown in Figure 110, two vertebral bodies were crossed with the fixator because the cranial vertebral body showed a longitudinal fissure fracture. Laminectomy was performed on the T 12 and L 1 vertebrae. After mobilization of the patient, an increase of kyphosis of 10° was observed on the postoperative radiograph after eight weeks, and an alteration in the position of the upper Schanz screws was evident. An ap radiograph showed that one of the screws did not converge towards the midline, but exited laterally from the pedicle and was situated beside the vertebral body. The patient refused further sur-

109

gery because he experienced a marked neurological recovery which he did not wish to endanger, and he was painfree. In the course of his rehabilitation, there was no further change in the position of the spine until the time of his discharge. The most recent radiograph available to us is six months post surgery. Shortly afterwards, the patient died of a pulmonary embolism from a femoroiliac vein thrombosis demonstrated at autopsy. At the time of autopsy, the fracture was consolidated, and there was no irritation or hematoma around the displaced screw in the connective tissue adjacent to the vertebral body.

Lateral positioning of the screw does not automatically lead to loss of correction, as shown by our second case. With similar positioning of the screw, complete anatomical reduction was maintained, as shown in Figure 70 in Section 8.5.

In the first patient of the entire series, lateral displacement of the fracture was inadequately reduced. The fixator rods took up a parallelogram shape, and finally consolidation occurred with the original displacement in the AP plane.

g) *Other:*

Occasionally on routine removal of the implant, the minor complication of fracture of one or two of the screws was seen in six patients where there was a solidly healed vertebral fracture (Fig. 111). In one case, the threaded rods were broken without any displacement (Fig. 112). These fractures do not have any functional significance. Usually the implant crosses at least one motion segment which is still capable of movement, and we deliberately aimed to avoid fusion at this level. Thus there is bound to be a flexion strain on the implant after fracture healing and in the long run this will lead to fatigue fracturing. It is desirable to preserve the mobility in the area which is instrumented. As a

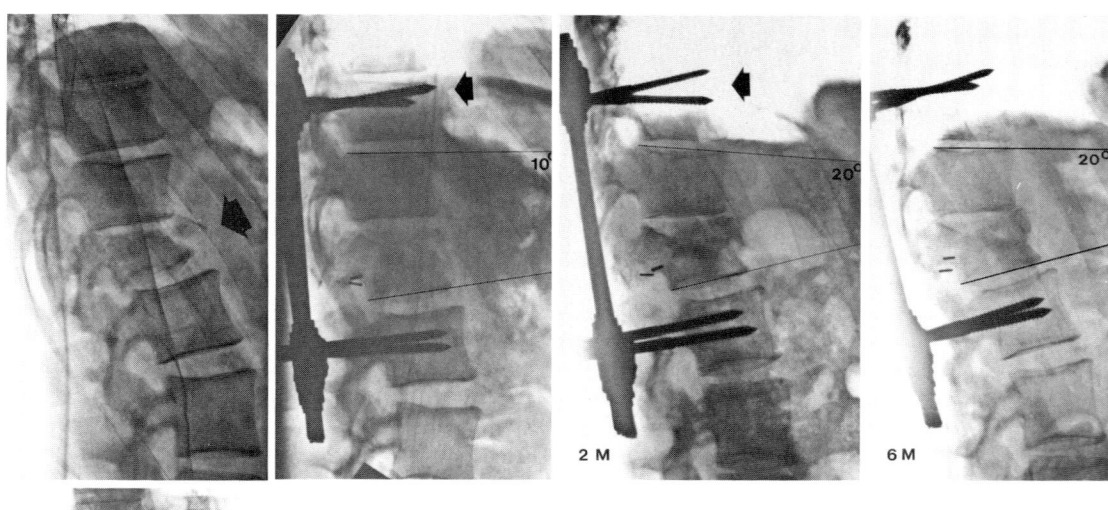

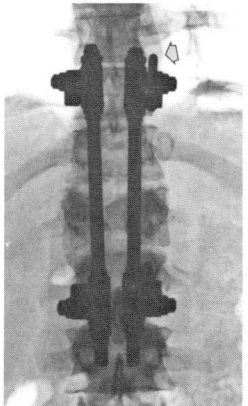

Fig. 110. After mobilization of this patient increase in kyphosis of 10°. Reasons for two level instrumentation are explained in the text. The ap radiograph shows that one of the upper screws has inadvertently been inserted laterally from the vertebral body (patient R.P., male, 29 years old).

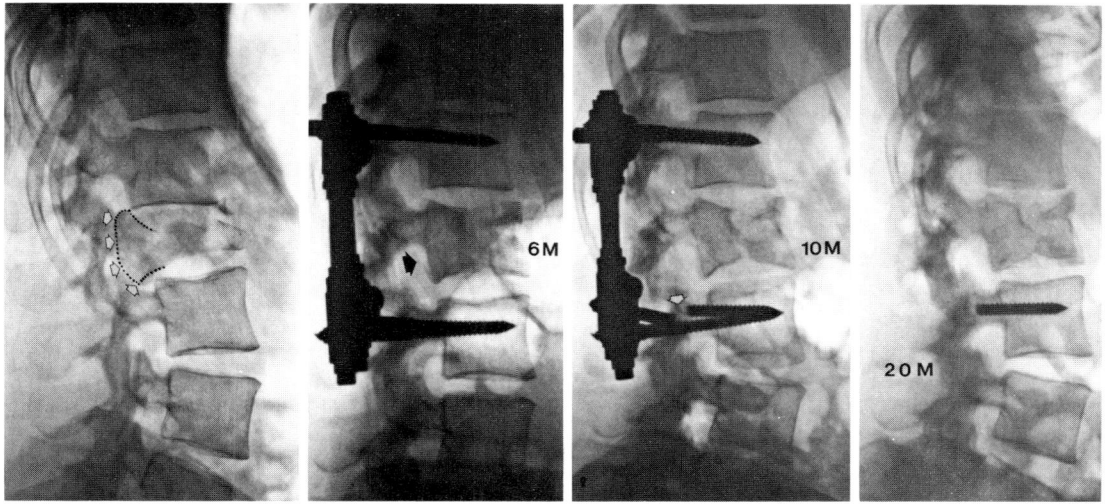

Fig. 111. Female patient early in the series: cancellous bone grafting was not carried out. Between the sixth and the tenth month after operation fatigue fracture of a Schanz screw without subjective symptoms (patient K.M., female, 28 years old).

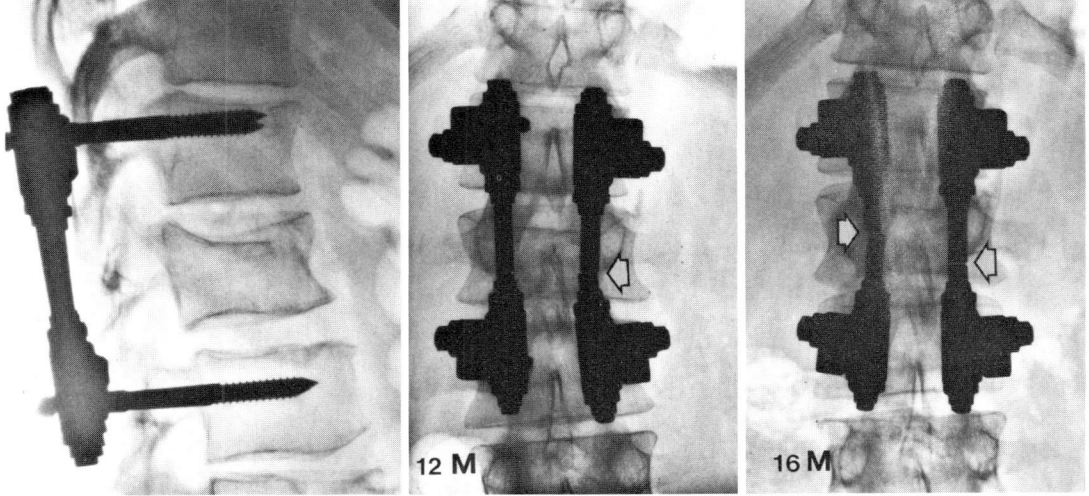

Fig. 112. This patient engaged in heavy manual work postponed implant removal for occupational reasons. After 12 months, a fatigue fracture occurred in one longitudinal rod, and after 16 months also in the other rod without displacement of the rods. Removal of the metal after 22 months (patient V.R., male, 27 years old).

result of this, it is important to fill any defects in the vertebral body in order to accelerate fracture healing, and it is also recommended that the implant is removed early, after eight to 12 months depending on the radiographic appearances.

There were six cases where there were either hematoma, delayed wound healing or superficial infections with fistulation. These did not delay early mobilization or normal fracture healing. In all cases, it was possible to remove the implant at the usual time and there were no further complications. Figure 113 shows an example.

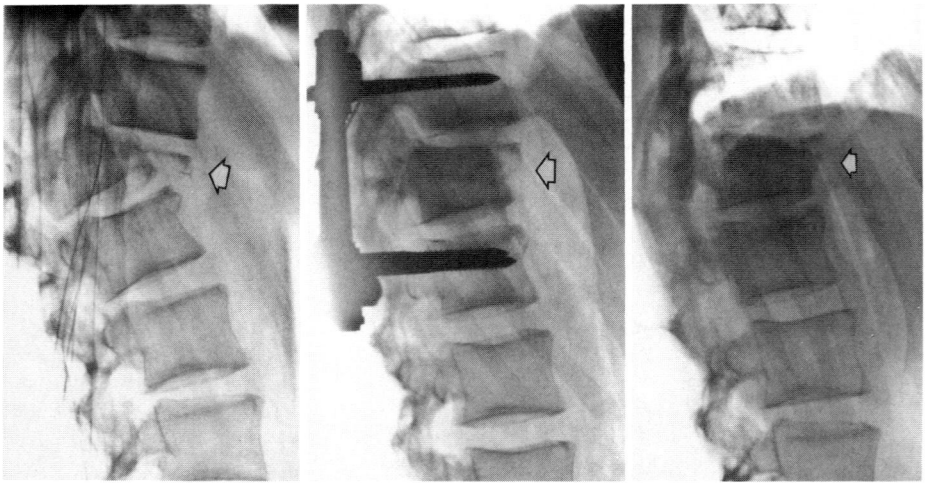

Fig. 113. T12/L1 fracture dislocation with complete disruption of the canal contents. Postoperative hematoma and wound dehiscence. Fistula formation, but undisturbed fracture consolidation. Implant removal after eight months, and 12 months later the wound was quiescent (patient M.L., male, 18 years old).

There were no vascular injuries among the 183 instrumentations. We were unable to detect any nerve root injury. With the exception of the group with severe spondylolisthesis, no neurological injury could be demonstrated in any patients.

h) *Neurological deficits in spondylolistheses:*

In the small group of 16 severe spondylolistheses, transient neurological deficits (namely hyperesthesia, paresthesia and pareses in the L4/S1 region) occurred in four cases as late as one to 10 days postoperatively. Direct damage to the nerve roots from the screws could be excluded due to the distribution of the nerve lesions. We attribute the neurological lesions to the substantial reduction. Most symptoms were only observed for a short period of time. Yet in one patient, the strength of the tibialis anterior muscle remained 0, in another patient 3 at nine months from surgery. All the patients were completely relieved of pain, and all stated at follow-up that they would still have undergone surgery despite the complications, due to the degree of improvement in daily life.

## 10.3 Discussion

The discussion should address itself to the clinical experience to date using the internal fixator for the treatment of vertebral fractures in the thoracolumbar spine, analysing the objectives for a new implant system designed to solve the problems cited in Section 6.1. Have these goals been achieved?

- *Fixation distance not more than two motion segments:* The bisegmental arthrodesis made possible using the internal fixator has clearly achieved this aim. During training for independence, all the patients noticed much better spinal mobility and this was of substantial functional value. The physiotherapists treating the patients knew from the function of the patients whether stabilization using Harrington distraction systems (or plates) or the internal fixator had been used. The five patients in whom a previous long fixation device had been replaced subsequently by an internal fixator lost their back symptoms and reported a subjective gain in function. In none of the patients to date has pain been observed during standing exercises with the necessary hyperextension of the spine. Pain is frequently reported in patients with long implants whilst doing this, as described by HASDAY et al. [73].

- *Versatility:* As demonstrated in Section 8, the internal fixator was used in various fracture forms with different biomechanical requirements. In various lesions with or without destruction of the posterior wall of the vertebral body, the dorsal columns, or the anterior longitudinal ligament, the fixator was used either in distraction, in compression or as a neutral fixation. Since it does not depend on any other bone structure apart from the vertebral bodies for fixation of the Schanz screws, different fracture types followed similar postoperative courses.

- *Fracture reduction:* The long lever arm of the Schanz screws is more suitable for reduction than all other implants with the exception of the external fixator. The internal fixator allows three dimensional movements due to the firm anchorage in bone, so that lordosis and kyphosis can be corrected. In very severe dislocations with major shortening, temporary use of a Harrington distraction rod may be recommended, when distraction of the spine requires very great force, which may compromise the fit of the Schanz screws if they are used for reduction. This was only necessary on two occasions early in this series.

- *Applicability after laminectomy:* In more than a dozen cases with prior laminectomy, we have shown that the fixator can be applied without technical problems. The Schanz screws are more easily placed due to the visualization of the dural canal. The remnants of the pedicles and the vertebral bodies are sufficient for stable anchoring of the screws.

- *Few special instruments and size graduations:* The bolt cutter for severing the projecting ends of the Schanz screws and two appropriate wrenches are the only special instruments required, apart from the instruments for anterior bone grafting as described in Sections 8.1 and 8.3.

  The implant has a uniform size which is merely extended by shorter or longer threaded rods for special applications.

- *Implantability; no additional external fixation:* Despite the volume of the implant, no particular difficulty has been found in wound closure. With regard to external support, we are still gaining experience cautiously. Until the end of the present series only tension band fixations and selected cooperative and reliable patients with fractures have received postoperative treatment without any external support. These comprise about one fifth of the reported cases. The remaining patients wore a three-point corset of the Jewett type for eight weeks postoperatively. Plaster casts or full contact corsets were not used. In 1987 postoperative treatment without external support was initiated as a standard procedure.

Thus the objectives have largely been achieved. In summary, it is clear that application of the internal fixator in fracture treatment requires excellent three dimensional conceptualization, anatomical knowledge and familiarity with a wide spectrum of other methods of stabilization and other operations by the surgeon. For this reason, the fixator should be used solely in surgical departments where the entire spectrum of spinal surgery is practiced. The principle of the internal fixator is short-distance fixation by pedicle screws which are connected in an angle-stable manner to a longitudinal load carrier. The fixator has proved to be successful both experimentally and clinically, and further development should be pursued as technical improvements are undoubtedly possible.

## 11. Appendix

More recently, much more detailed experimental measurements have become available from WÖRSDÖRFER [216] and KORTMANN [98]. These measurements include torsional forces and encompass a series of other implants. The results confirm the evaluations in Sections 4–7 using our own measurements on the internal fixator.

For the experiments in Section 7, a universal materials testing machine (Rumul Mikrotron 654) was used. This allows measurements of continuously rising or falling loads which are applied via a spindle drive. The load can be measured using a built-in load measuring device.

Two inductive goniometers (Schaevitz RVDT type R 30 A, Schaevitz, Pennsauken, New Jersey, USA) are used to measure angular deformity. The measurement range is ± 40° with a precision of ± 0.5%. Two goniometers were screwed into the anterior aspect of the vertebral bodies, cranially and caudally to the lesion. Thus the alteration in angle between the two vertebrae

gave the angular deformation between the two goniometers in the injured area during flexion stress (Fig. 114).

When the load measuring device moves upwards via the spindle drive, there is a distally directed traction force exerted on the ventral part of the 360 mm long stirrup screwed on to the specimen with an equally large countertraction in proximal direction at the dorsal end of the stirrup. If the angulation of the spine increases, the roller carriage with ball and socket anchoring can roll forward, and thus avoid additional shearing forces.

The goniometers, load measuring device, amplifier and plotter were calibrated with precision angle meters and calibration weights and adjusted to a defined paper feed. For evaluation, the difference between the two goniometer curves in relation to the load was measured manually in 5 mm steps on the x axis after compensation for parallax. The digital figures were read into a computer (Nova III, Data General) and incorporated into tables, with simultaneous calculation of the flexion moment M in accordance with the formula

$$M = \frac{F \cdot d}{2}$$

d is a constant of 360 mm corresponding to the length of the stirrup screwed on to the specimen, resulting in the uneven values for the flexion moment in Nm in the following tables (the printout with five decimal places after the point is due to the computer and is not a reflection on the precision of measurement).

The angulation deformities were represented via computer in relation to the flexion moment for the individual trial courses on a printer plotter (Printronix P 300) with a plot program of our own. As usual, the flexion moment was plotted on the y axis and the angular deformation on the x axis.

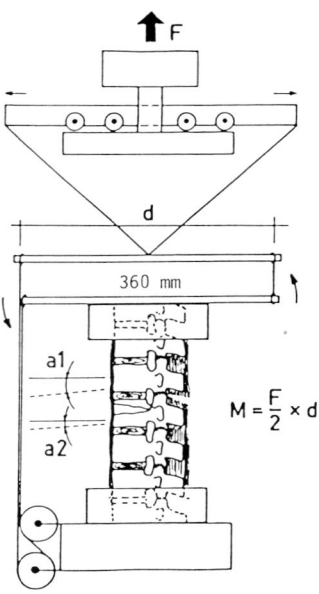

Fig. 114. Experimental setting described by WÖRSDÖRFER [214] for application of pure flexion moment M to the spinal specimen. The deformation of the injured segment is determined by goniometers on a1 and a2, established by the difference between their measured values. d = 360 mm.

## Experimental results for Section 7.1. Elastic and plastic deformation.

Table 5

| Flexion moment Nm | distance a with increasing flexion moment mm | distance a with decreasing flexion moment (hysteresis) mm |
|---|---|---|
| . 00000 | . 00000 | . 00000 |
| 1. 25000 | . 19800 | . 37950 |
| 2. 50000 | . 41250 | . 74250 |
| 3. 75000 | . 57750 | . 99000 |
| 5. 00000 | . 74250 | 1. 23750 |
| 6. 25000 | . 92400 | 1. 48500 |
| 7. 50000 | 1. 12200 | 1. 68300 |
| 8. 75000 | 1. 28700 | 1. 91400 |
| 10. 00000 | 1. 45200 | 2. 07900 |
| 11. 25000 | 1. 61700 | 2. 21100 |
| 12. 50000 | 1. 78200 | 2. 39250 |
| 13. 75000 | 1. 94700 | 2. 50800 |
| 15. 00000 | 2. 11200 | 2. 64000 |
| 16. 25000 | 2. 27700 | 2. 77200 |
| 17. 50000 | 2. 44200 | 2. 87100 |
| 18. 75000 | 2. 60700 | 3. 00300 |
| 20. 00000 | 2. 77200 | 3. 10200 |
| 21. 25000 | 2. 93700 | 3. 20100 |
| 22. 50000 | 3. 10200 | 3. 33300 |
| 23. 75000 | 3. 26700 | 3. 39900 |
| 25. 00000 | 3. 43200 | 3. 43200 |

Table 6

| Flexion moment Nm | distance a with increasing flexion moment mm | distance a with decreasing flexion moment (hysteresis) mm |
|---|---|---|
| . 00000 | . 00000 | . 00000 |
| 1. 25000 | . 19800 | . 42900 |
| 2. 50000 | . 41250 | . 82500 |
| 3. 75000 | . 57750 | 1. 08900 |
| 5. 00000 | . 74250 | 1. 35300 |
| 6. 25000 | . 92400 | 1. 61700 |
| 7. 50000 | 1. 12200 | 1. 84800 |
| 8. 75000 | 1. 28700 | 2. 11200 |
| 10. 00000 | 1. 45200 | 2. 31000 |
| 11. 25000 | 1. 61700 | 2. 47500 |
| 12. 50000 | 1. 78200 | 2. 57400 |
| 13. 75000 | 1. 94700 | 2. 77200 |
| 15. 00000 | 2. 11200 | 2. 90400 |
| 16. 25000 | 2. 27700 | 3. 03600 |
| 17. 50000 | 2. 44200 | 3. 16800 |
| 18. 75000 | 2. 60700 | 3. 30000 |
| 20. 00000 | 2. 77200 | 3. 43200 |
| 21. 25000 | 2. 93700 | 3. 51450 |
| 22. 50000 | 3. 10200 | 3. 63000 |
| 23. 75000 | 3. 26700 | 3. 76200 |
| 25. 00000 | 3. 43200 | 3. 86100 |
| 26. 25000 | 3. 59700 | 3. 96000 |
| 27. 50000 | 3. 76200 | 4. 09200 |
| 28. 75000 | 3. 92700 | 4. 19100 |
| 30. 00000 | 4. 05900 | 4. 29000 |
| 31. 25000 | 4. 21080 | 4. 37250 |
| 32. 50000 | 4. 37250 | 4. 48800 |
| 33. 75000 | 4. 50450 | 4. 60350 |
| 35. 00000 | 4. 66950 | 4. 66950 |

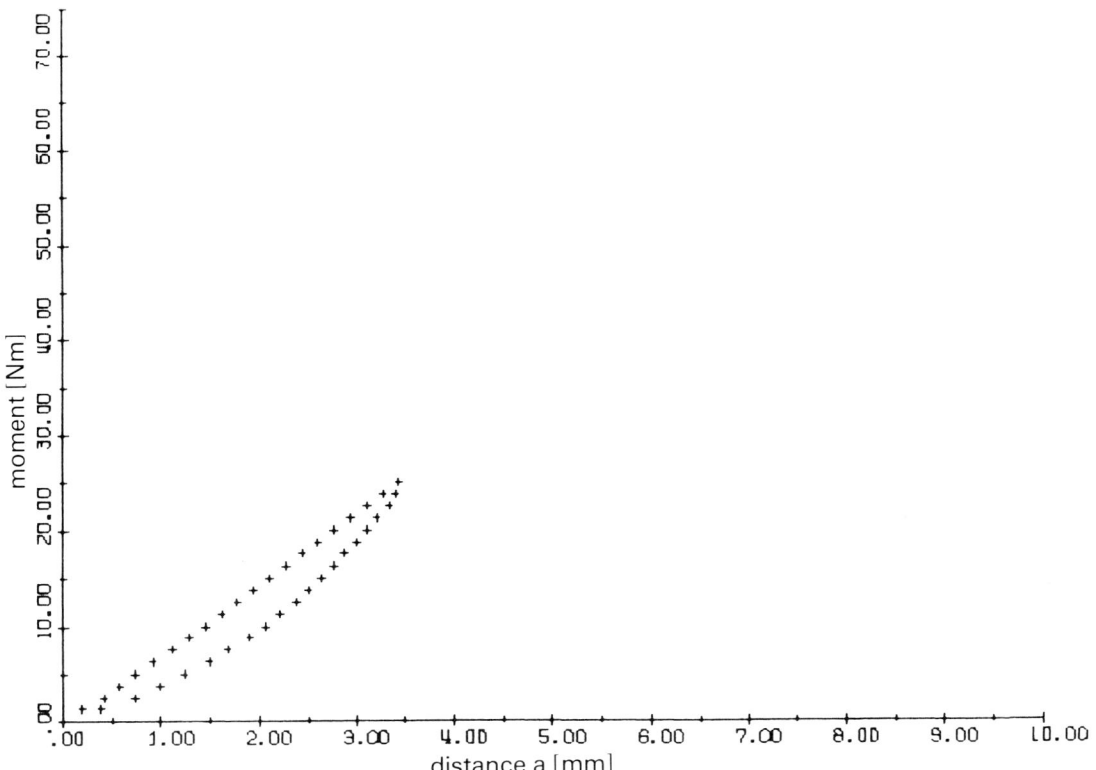

Fig. 115

115

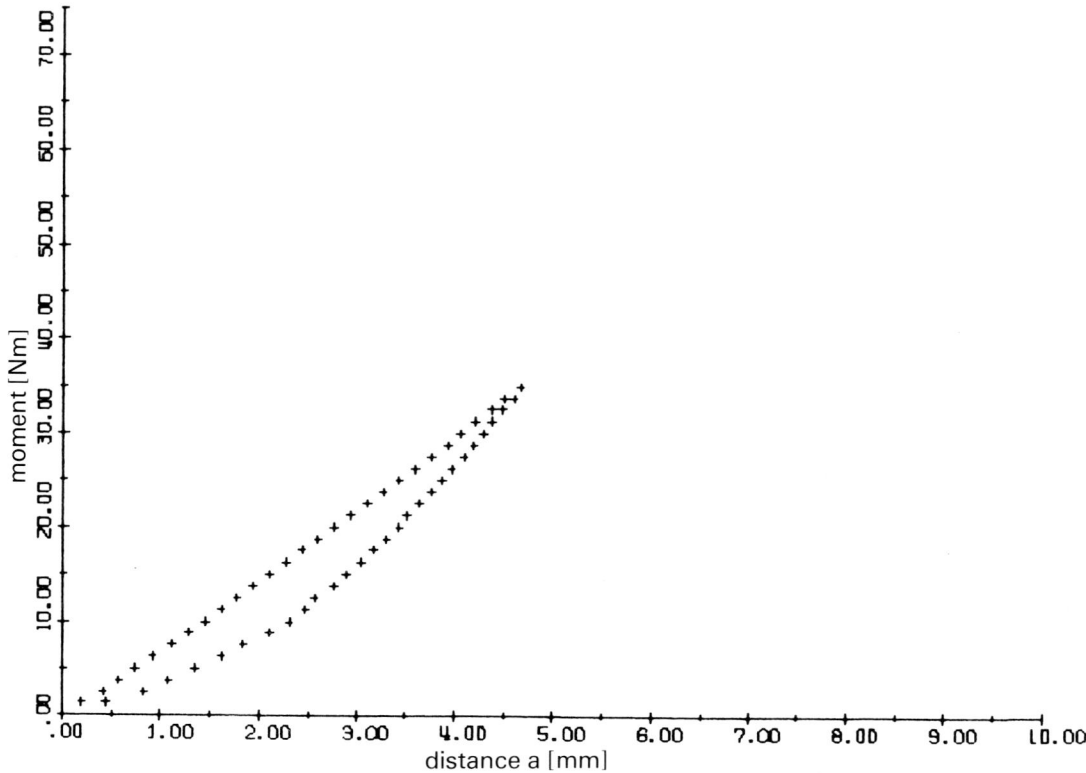

Fig. 116

Table 7

| Flexion moment Nm | distance a with increasing flexion moment mm | distance a with decreasing flexion moment (hysteresis) mm |
|---|---|---|
| .00000 | .00000 | .16500 |
| 1.25000 | .19800 | .56100 |
| 2.50000 | .41250 | .89100 |
| 3.75000 | .57750 | 1.15500 |
| 5.00000 | .74250 | 1.45200 |
| 6.25000 | .92400 | 1.71600 |
| 7.50000 | 1.12200 | 1.98000 |
| 8.75000 | 1.28700 | 2.24400 |
| 10.00000 | 1.45200 | 2.44200 |
| 11.25000 | 1.61700 | 2.60700 |
| 12.50000 | 1.78200 | 2.73900 |
| 13.75000 | 1.94700 | 2.87100 |
| 15.00000 | 2.11200 | 3.03600 |
| 16.25000 | 2.27700 | 3.16800 |
| 17.50000 | 2.44200 | 3.30000 |
| 18.75000 | 2.60700 | 3.43200 |
| 20.00000 | 2.77200 | 3.56400 |
| 21.25000 | 2.93700 | 3.66300 |
| 22.50000 | 3.10200 | 3.79500 |
| 23.75000 | 3.26700 | 3.92700 |
| 25.00000 | 3.43200 | 4.05900 |
| 26.25000 | 3.59700 | 4.15800 |
| 27.50000 | 3.76200 | 4.29000 |
| 28.75000 | 3.92700 | 4.37250 |
| 30.00000 | 4.05900 | 4.48800 |
| 31.25000 | 4.20750 | 4.62000 |
| 32.50000 | 4.37250 | 4.71900 |
| 33.75000 | 4.50450 | 4.81800 |
| 35.00000 | 4.66950 | 4.91700 |
| 36.25000 | 4.75200 | 5.01600 |
| 37.50000 | 4.90050 | 5.13150 |
| 38.75000 | 5.03250 | 5.21400 |
| 40.00000 | 5.16450 | 5.32950 |
| 41.25000 | 5.31300 | 5.41200 |
| 42.50000 | 5.46150 | 5.46150 |

116

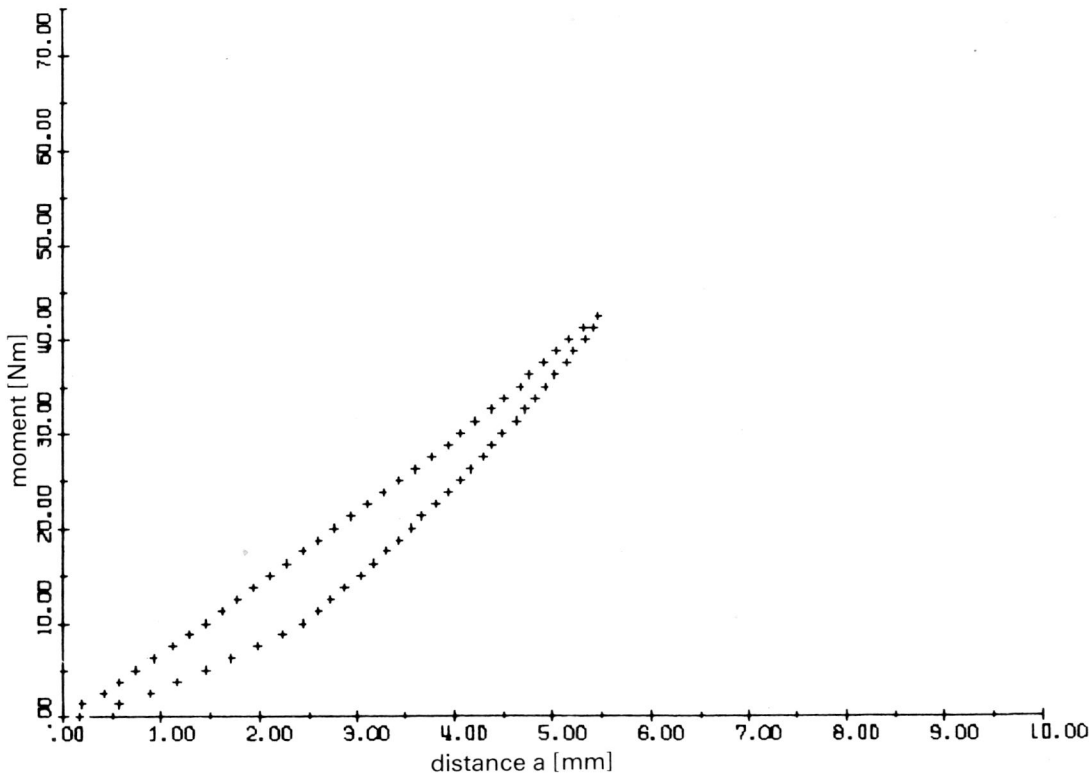

Fig. 117

Experimental results for Section 7.2.2. Deformation in the fracture model.

Spine 1: no. 285/83; female, 83 years old.

Table 8. Angular deformation between L1 and L3 relative to the flexion moment in the intact spine, after experimental combined anterior and posterior lesion of L2 and after instrumentation with internal fixator L1–L3.

S 1

| Flexion moment [Nm] | Angular deformity intact spine [degrees] | lesion [degrees] | Internal fixator [degrees] |
|---|---|---|---|
| .36000 | .70000 | 4.20000 | .00000 |
| .72000 | 1.50000 | 6.40000 | .05000 |
| 1.08000 | 2.20000 | 7.90000 | .10000 |
| 1.44000 | 2.80000 | 8.90000 | .10000 |
| 1.80000 | 3.40000 | 9.90000 | .20000 |
| 2.16000 | 3.90000 | 10.60000 | .40000 |
| 2.52000 | 4.20000 | 11.30000 | .40000 |
| 2.88000 | 4.60000 | 11.90000 | .50000 |
| 3.24000 | 4.90000 | 12.70000 | .60000 |
| 3.60000 | 5.10000 | 13.40000 | .70000 |
| 3.96000 | 5.30000 | 13.90000 | .85000 |
| 4.32000 | 5.40000 | 14.40000 | .95000 |
| 4.68000 | 5.45000 | 15.20000 | 1.10000 |
| 5.04000 | 5.50000 | 15.70000 | 1.20000 |
| 5.40000 | 5.55000 | 16.20000 | 1.30000 |
| 5.76000 | 5.65000 | | 1.40000 |
| 6.12000 | 5.70000 | | 1.60000 |
| 6.48000 | 5.80000 | | 1.75000 |
| 6.84000 | 5.95000 | | 1.95000 |
| 7.20000 | 6.10000 | | 2.10000 |
| 7.56000 | 6.15000 | | 2.30000 |
| 7.92000 | 6.25000 | | 2.45000 |
| 8.28000 | 6.30000 | | 2.70000 |
| 8.64000 | 6.40000 | | 2.90000 |
| 9.00000 | 6.50000 | | 3.20000 |

S 1

| Flexion moment [Nm] | Angular deformity intact spine [degrees] | lesion [degrees] | Internal fixator [degrees] |
|---|---|---|---|
| 9.36000 | 6.60000 | | 3.40000 |
| 9.72000 | 6.65000 | | 3.70000 |
| 10.08000 | 6.70000 | | 3.90000 |
| 10.44000 | 6.80000 | | 4.10000 |
| 10.80000 | 6.85000 | | 4.40000 |
| 11.52000 | 7.00000 | | 4.80000 |
| 12.24000 | 7.25000 | | 5.20000 |
| 12.96000 | 7.40000 | | 5.50000 |
| 13.68000 | 7.55000 | | 5.90000 |
| 14.40000 | 7.70000 | | 6.30000 |
| 15.12000 | 7.80000 | | 6.70000 |
| 15.84000 | 7.90000 | | 7.30000 |
| 16.56000 | 8.05000 | | 7.60000 |
| 17.28000 | 8.15000 | | 7.95000 |
| 18.00000 | 8.30000 | | 8.30000 |
| 18.71999 | 8.40000 | | 8.60000 |
| 19.43999 | | | 9.10000 |
| 20.15999 | | | 9.40000 |
| 20.87999 | | | 9.70000 |
| 21.59999 | | | 10.00000 |
| 22.31999 | | | 10.20000 |
| 23.03999 | | | 10.50000 |
| 23.75999 | | | 10.70000 |
| 24.48000 | | | 11.00000 |
| 25.20000 | | | 11.20000 |

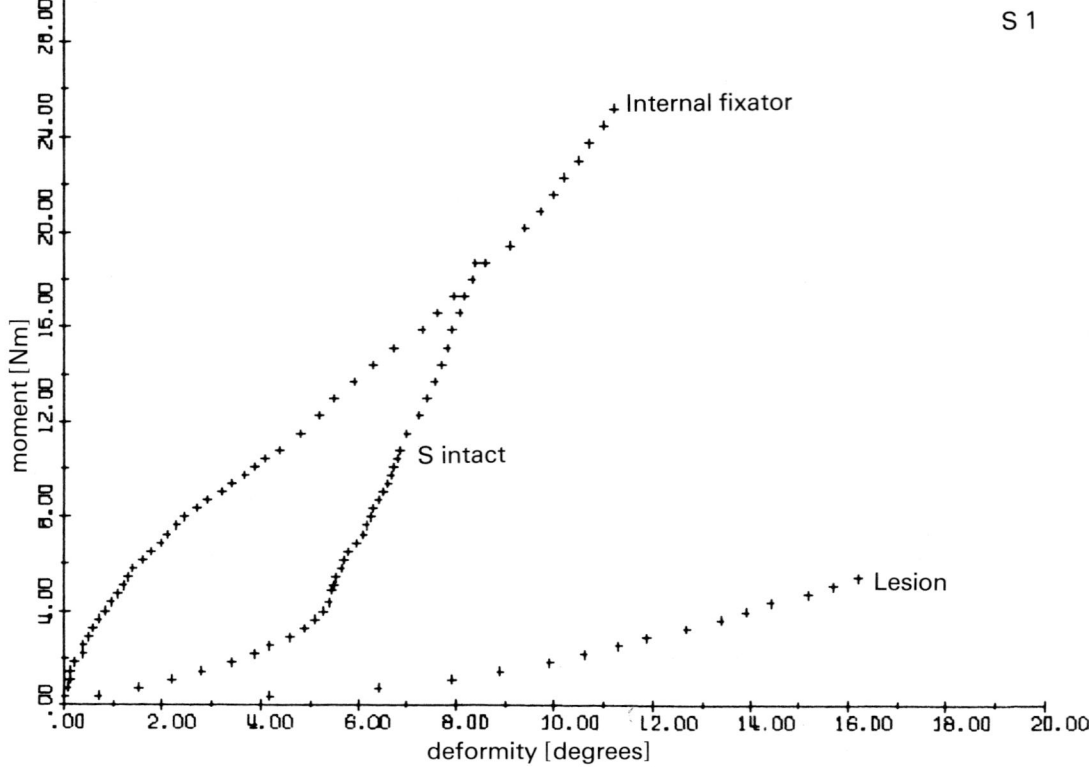

Fig. 118. Specimen S1. Angular deformity in degrees between L1 and L3 before and after fracture created at L2 with anterior and posterior instability. The diagram shows the figures for the intact spine, the fractured spine and the fractured spine with the internal fixator, submitted to a pure flexion moment. Measurements are in Nm (ordinate).

## Spine 2: no. 284/83; female, 83 years old.

Table 9. Specimen S2

S 2

| Flexion moment [Nm] | Angular deformity intact spine [degrees] | lesion [degrees] | Internal fixator [degrees] |
|---|---|---|---|
| .36000 | 1.10000 | 1.90000 | .10000 |
| .72000 | 2.20000 | 3.80000 | .20000 |
| 1.08000 | 3.00000 | 5.10000 | .20000 |
| 1.44000 | 3.60000 | 6.00000 | .30000 |
| 1.80000 | 4.10000 | 6.90000 | .30000 |
| 2.16000 | 4.50000 | 7.50000 | .40000 |
| 2.52000 | 4.90000 | 7.90000 | .50000 |
| 2.88000 | 5.20000 | 8.40000 | .60000 |
| 3.24000 | 5.50000 | 8.80000 | .65000 |
| 3.60000 | 5.70000 | 9.10000 | .75000 |
| 3.96000 | 5.90000 | 9.40000 | .80000 |
| 4.32000 | 6.10000 | 9.70000 | .90000 |
| 4.68000 | 6.40000 | 10.00000 | .95000 |
| 5.04000 | 6.50000 | 10.20000 | 1.00000 |
| 5.40000 | 6.60000 | 10.40000 | 1.10000 |
| 5.76000 | 6.80000 | 10.70000 | 1.20000 |
| 6.12000 | 6.90000 | 10.80000 | 1.20000 |
| 6.48000 | 7.00000 | 11.00000 | 1.30000 |
| 6.84000 | 7.10000 | 11.20000 | 1.40000 |
| 7.20000 | 7.30000 | 11.40000 | 1.45000 |
| 7.56000 | 7.40000 | 11.50000 | 1.55000 |
| 7.92000 | 7.40000 | 11.70000 | 1.65000 |
| 8.28000 | 7.50000 | 11.80000 | 1.75000 |
| 8.64000 | 7.60000 | 12.00000 | 1.80000 |
| 9.00000 | 7.70000 | 12.10000 | 1.90000 |

S 2

| Flexion moment [Nm] | Angular deformity intact spine [degrees] | lesion [degrees] | Internal fixator [degrees] |
|---|---|---|---|
| 9.36000 | 7.80000 | 12.30000 | 2.00000 |
| 9.72000 | 7.80000 | 12.40000 | 2.10000 |
| 10.08000 | 7.80000 | 12.50000 | 2.20000 |
| 10.44000 | 7.90000 | 12.70000 | 2.30000 |
| 10.80000 | 7.90000 | 12.80000 | 2.35000 |
| 11.52000 | 8.00000 | 13.10000 | 2.60000 |
| 12.24000 | 8.10000 | 13.20000 | 2.80000 |
| 12.96000 | 8.20000 | 13.30000 | 3.00000 |
| 13.68000 | 8.40000 | 13.50000 | 3.20000 |
| 14.40000 | 8.60000 | | 3.40000 |
| 15.12000 | 8.70000 | | 3.60000 |
| 15.84000 | 8.80000 | | 3.80000 |
| 16.56000 | 8.90000 | | 4.00000 |
| 17.28000 | 9.10000 | | 4.20000 |
| 18.00000 | 9.30000 | | 4.35000 |
| 18.71999 | 9.40000 | | 4.50000 |
| 19.43999 | 9.50000 | | 4.70000 |
| 20.15999 | 9.60000 | | 4.90000 |
| 20.87999 | | | 5.10000 |
| 21.59999 | | | 5.30000 |
| 22.31999 | | | 5.50000 |
| 23.03999 | | | 5.70000 |
| 23.75999 | | | 5.90000 |
| 24.48000 | | | 6.10000 |

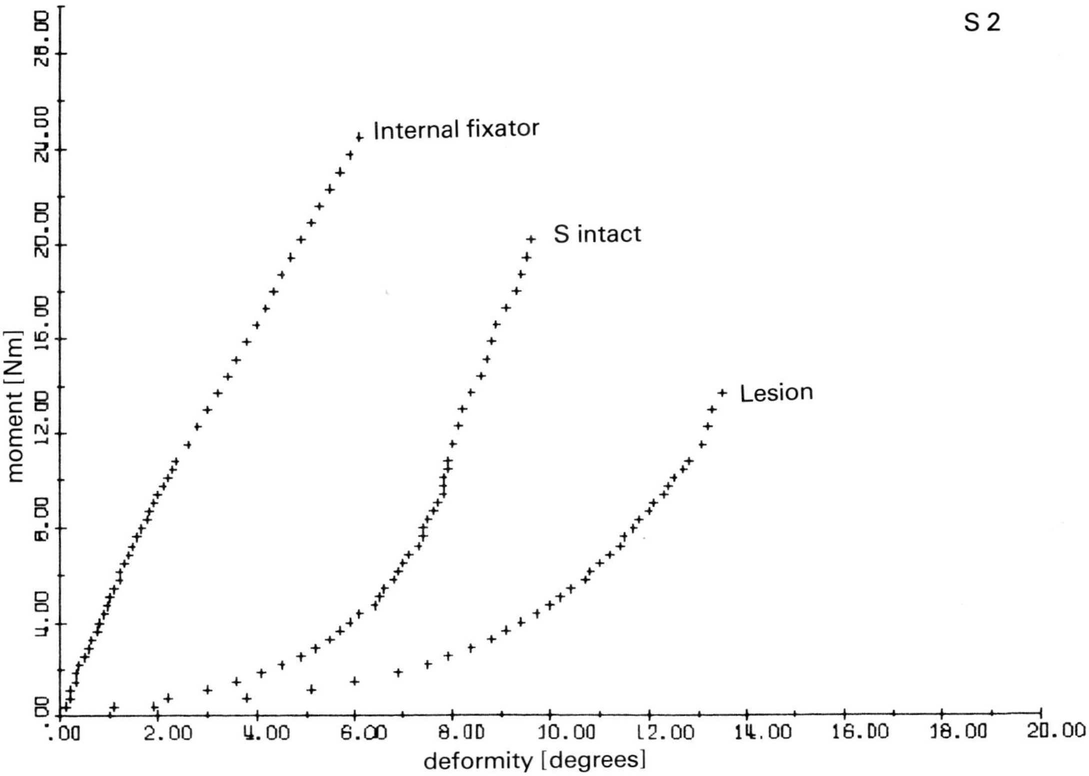

Fig. 119. Specimen S2

This specimen showed the least autolytic changes. It was submitted to 47,5 Nm in a second test run. After unloading, there remained a residual plastic deformation of 0.3 degrees.

Table 10. Specimen S2. Second test run with higher flexion moments applied to the instrumented spine.

S 2

| Flexion moment [Nm] | Angular deformity intact spine [degrees] | lesion [degrees] | Internal fixator [degrees] |
|---|---|---|---|
| . 72000 | | | . 10000 |
| 1. 44000 | | | . 30000 |
| 2. 16000 | | | . 45000 |
| 2. 88000 | | | . 60000 |
| 3. 60000 | | | . 80000 |
| 4. 32000 | | | . 90000 |
| 5. 04000 | | | 1. 05000 |
| 5. 76000 | | | 1. 20000 |
| 6. 48000 | | | 1. 40000 |
| 7. 20000 | | | 1. 50000 |
| 7. 92000 | | | 1. 70000 |
| 8. 64000 | | | 1. 85000 |
| 9. 36000 | | | 2. 00000 |
| 10. 08000 | | | 2. 20000 |
| 10. 80000 | | | 2. 45000 |
| 11. 52000 | | | 2. 60000 |
| 12. 24000 | | | 2. 80000 |
| 12. 96000 | | | 3. 00000 |
| 13. 68000 | | | 3. 20000 |
| 14. 40000 | | | 3. 40000 |
| 15. 12000 | | | 3. 55000 |
| 15. 84000 | | | 3. 70000 |
| 16. 55998 | | | 3. 85000 |
| 17. 27998 | | | 4. 00000 |

S 2

| Flexion moment [Nm] | Angular deformity intact spine [degrees] | lesion [degrees] | Internal fixator [degrees] |
|---|---|---|---|
| 17. 99998 | | | 4. 20000 |
| 18. 71999 | | | 4. 40000 |
| 19. 43999 | | | 4. 50000 |
| 20. 15999 | | | 4. 70000 |
| 20. 87999 | | | 4. 90000 |
| 21. 59999 | | | 5. 10000 |
| 23. 03999 | | | 5. 40000 |
| 24. 47998 | | | 5. 70000 |
| 25. 91998 | | | 6. 00000 |
| 27. 35999 | | | 6. 20000 |
| 28. 79999 | | | 6. 40000 |
| 30. 23999 | | | 6. 60000 |
| 31. 67998 | | | 6. 85000 |
| 33. 11998 | | | 7. 15000 |
| 34. 55998 | | | 7. 35000 |
| 35. 99998 | | | 7. 60000 |
| 37. 43999 | | | 7. 80000 |
| 38. 87997 | | | 8. 00000 |
| 40. 31998 | | | 8. 20000 |
| 41. 75998 | | | 8. 40000 |
| 43. 19998 | | | 8. 60000 |
| 44. 63998 | | | 8. 70000 |
| 46. 07999 | | | 8. 90000 |
| 47. 51997 | | | 9. 10000 |

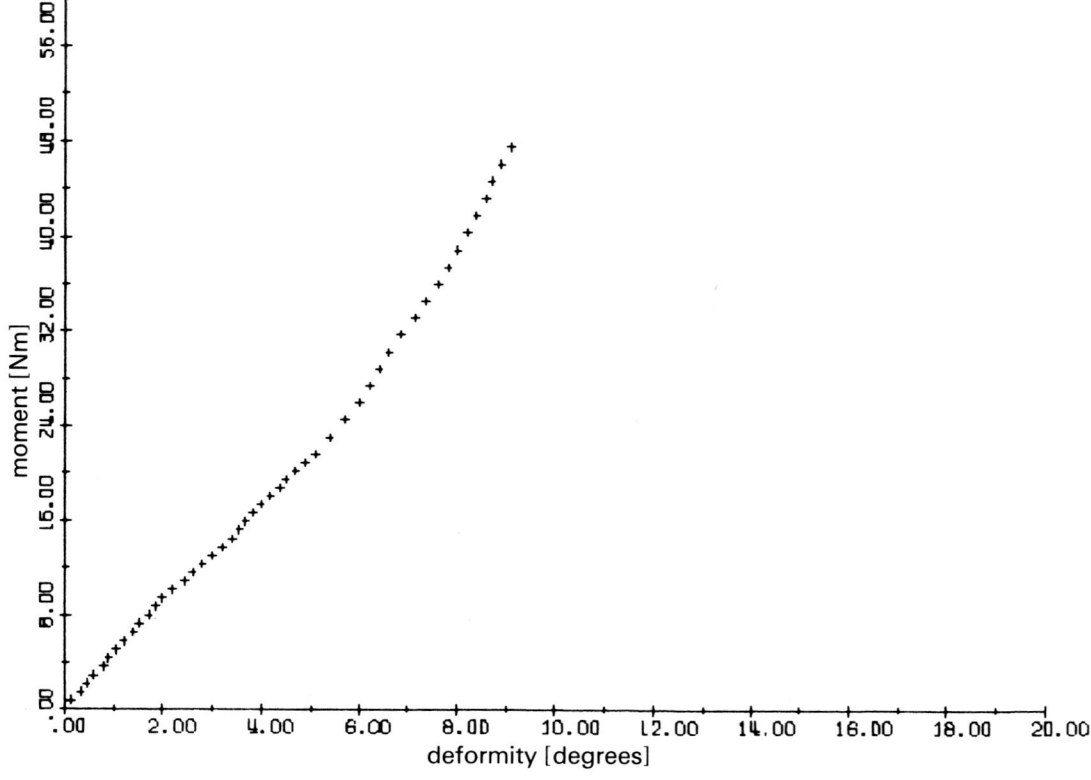

Fig. 120. Specimen S2. Second test run with internal fixator. Scale of the ordinate altered!

Spine 3: no. 463/83; male, 67 years old.

Table 11. Specimen S3

S 3

| Flexion moment [Nm] | Angular deformity intact spine [degrees] | lesion [degrees] | Internal fixator [degrees] |
|---|---|---|---|
| .72000 | .20000 | 2.90000 | .20000 |
| 1.44000 | .50000 | 6.10000 | .40000 |
| 2.16000 | 1.00000 | 8.40000 | .50000 |
| 2.88000 | 1.70000 | 10.10000 | .80000 |
| 3.60000 | 2.50000 | 11.70000 | 1.00000 |
| 4.32000 | 3.20000 | 12.60000 | 1.40000 |
| 5.04000 | 3.70000 | 13.40000 | 1.80000 |
| 5.76000 | 4.00000 | 13.90000 | 2.10000 |
| 6.48000 | 4.20000 | 14.30000 | 2.50000 |
| 7.20000 | 4.60000 | | 2.90000 |
| 7.92000 | 5.00000 | | 3.40000 |
| 8.64000 | 5.20000 | | 3.90000 |
| 9.36000 | 5.40000 | | 4.50000 |
| 10.08000 | 5.60000 | | 5.10000 |
| 10.80000 | 5.90000 | | 5.80000 |
| 11.52000 | 6.10000 | | 6.40000 |
| 12.24000 | 6.20000 | | 6.80000 |
| 12.96000 | 6.40000 | | 7.30000 |
| 13.68000 | 6.50000 | | 7.90000 |
| 14.40000 | 6.60000 | | 8.40000 |
| 15.12000 | 6.70000 | | 8.90000 |
| 15.84000 | 6.75000 | | 9.20000 |
| 16.55998 | 6.80000 | | 9.60000 |
| | | | 10.30000 |

S 3

| Flexion moment [Nm] | Angular deformity intact spine [degrees] | lesion [degrees] | Internal fixator [degrees] |
|---|---|---|---|
| 17.27998 | 6.90000 | | |
| 17.99998 | 7.00000 | | |
| 18.71999 | 7.10000 | | |
| 19.43999 | 7.25000 | | |
| 20.15999 | 7.30000 | | |
| 20.87999 | 7.40000 | | |
| 21.59999 | 7.50000 | | |
| 23.03999 | 7.70000 | | |
| 24.47998 | 7.90000 | | |
| 25.91998 | 8.00000 | | |
| 27.35999 | 8.20000 | | |
| 28.79999 | 8.30000 | | |
| 30.23999 | 8.40000 | | |
| 31.67998 | 8.60000 | | |
| 33.11998 | 8.70000 | | |
| 34.55998 | 8.80000 | | |
| 35.99998 | 8.90000 | | |
| 37.43999 | 9.00000 | | |
| 38.87997 | 9.10000 | | |
| 40.31998 | 9.10000 | | |
| 41.75998 | 9.20000 | | |
| 43.19998 | 9.30000 | | |

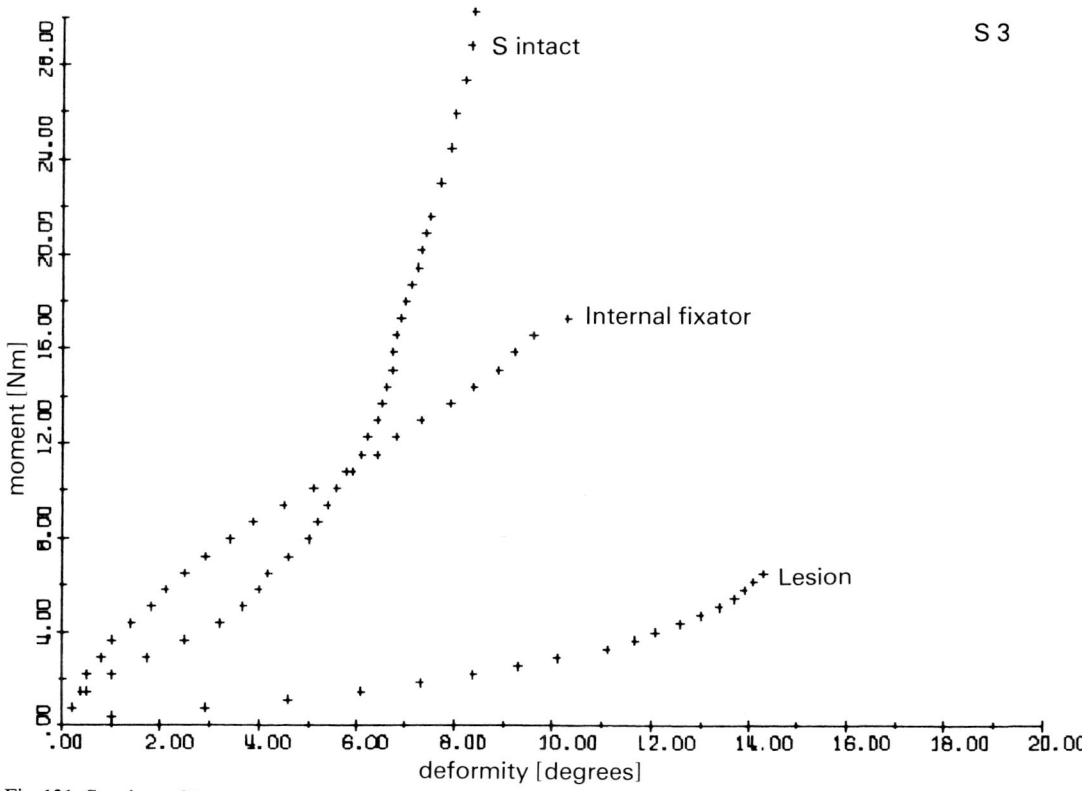

Fig. 121. Specimen S3

When the flexion moment exceeded 10 Nm, there was a slow giving way of the cancellous bone around the Schanz screws.

Spine 4: no. 288/83; female, 83 years old.

Table 12. Specimen S4

S 4

| Flexion moment [Nm] | Angular deformity intact spine [degrees] | lesion [degrees] | Internal fixator [degrees] |
|---|---|---|---|
| .72000 | 2.40000 | 5.60000 | .30000 |
| 1.44000 | 4.00000 | 9.10000 | .40000 |
| 2.16000 | 4.90000 | 11.00000 | .50000 |
| 2.88000 | 5.70000 | 12.00000 | .80000 |
| 3.60000 | 5.90000 | 12.80000 | .90000 |
| 4.32000 | 6.30000 | 13.40000 | 1.00000 |
| 5.04000 | 6.60000 | 14.10000 | 1.20000 |
| 5.76000 | 7.20000 | | 1.40000 |
| 6.48000 | 7.70000 | | 1.70000 |
| 7.20000 | 7.90000 | | 1.90000 |
| 7.92000 | 8.10000 | | 2.20000 |
| 8.64000 | 8.60000 | | 2.60000 |
| 9.36000 | 8.90000 | | 3.00000 |
| 10.08000 | 9.20000 | | 3.40000 |
| 10.80000 | 9.30000 | | 3.90000 |
| 11.52000 | 9.50000 | | 4.70000 |
| 12.24000 | 9.70000 | | 5.50000 |
| 12.96000 | 9.90000 | | 6.40000 |

S 4

| Flexion moment [Nm] | Angular deformity intact spine [degrees] | lesion [degrees] | Internal fixator [degrees] |
|---|---|---|---|
| 13.68000 | 9.90000 | | 7.30000 |
| 14.40000 | 9.90000 | | 8.60000 |
| 15.12000 | 9.90000 | | 9.90000 |
| 15.84000 | 10.00000 | | 10.90000 |
| 16.55998 | | | 12.10000 |
| 17.27998 | | | 13.20000 |
| 17.99998 | | | 14.50000 |
| 18.71999 | | | 15.20000 |
| 19.43999 | | | 16.20000 |
| 20.15999 | | | 17.00000 |
| 20.87999 | | | 17.89999 |
| 21.59999 | | | 18.60001 |

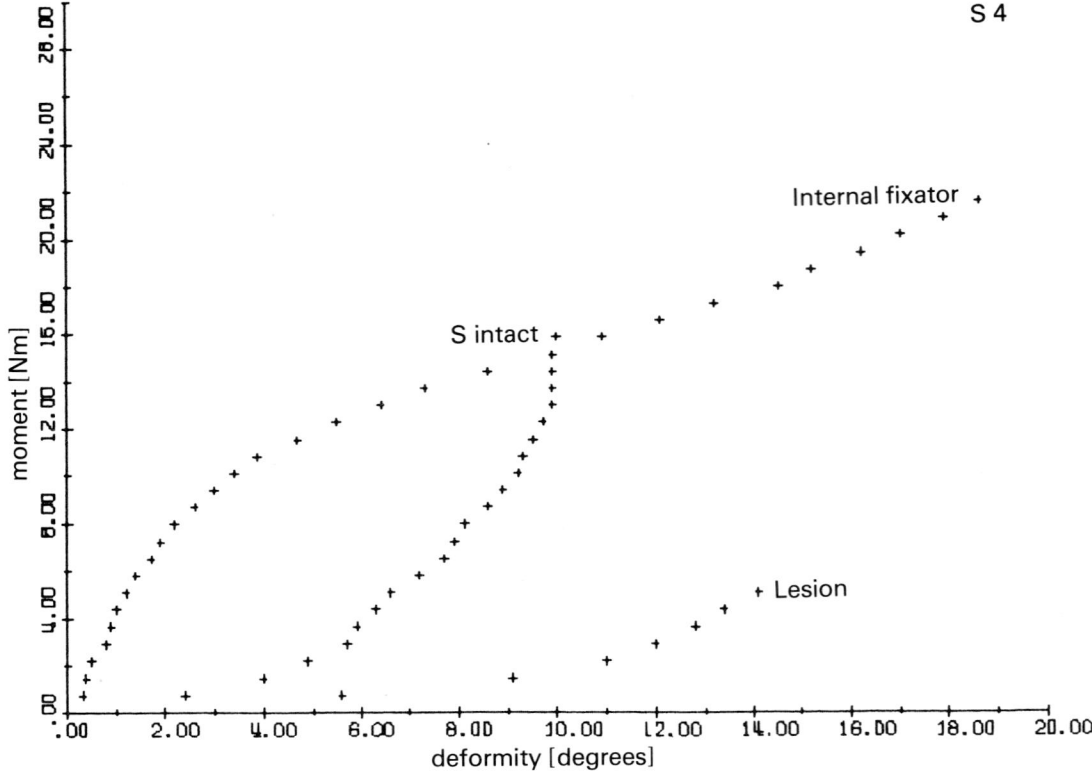

Fig. 122. Specimen S4

Spine 5: no. 462/83; male, 74 years old.

Table 13. Specimen S5

S 5

| Flexion moment [Nm] | Angular deformity | | Internal fixator [degrees] |
|---|---|---|---|
| | intact spine [degrees] | lesion [degrees] | |
| . 36000 | . 30000 | 5. 00000 | . 00000 |
| . 72000 | . 70000 | 6. 10000 | . 00000 |
| 1. 08000 | 1. 10000 | 6. 70000 | . 00000 |
| 1. 44000 | 1. 40000 | 7. 50000 | . 20000 |
| 1. 80000 | 1. 70000 | 8. 00000 | . 30000 |
| 2. 16000 | 2. 00000 | 8. 30000 | . 40000 |
| 2. 52000 | 2. 20000 | 8. 60000 | . 50000 |
| 2. 88000 | 2. 35000 | 8. 80000 | . 60000 |
| 3. 24000 | 2. 50000 | 9. 10000 | . 70000 |
| 3. 60000 | 2. 70000 | 9. 30000 | . 80000 |
| 3. 96000 | 2. 90000 | 9. 50000 | . 85000 |
| 4. 32000 | 3. 00000 | 9. 80000 | . 90000 |
| 4. 68000 | 3. 10000 | 10. 00000 | 1. 05000 |
| 5. 04000 | 3. 20000 | 10. 20000 | 1. 10000 |
| 5. 40000 | 3. 20000 | 10. 30000 | 1. 20000 |
| 5. 76000 | 3. 20000 | 10. 50000 | 1. 30000 |
| 6. 12000 | 3. 20000 | 10. 60000 | 1. 40000 |
| 6. 48000 | 3. 30000 | 10. 70000 | 1. 55000 |
| 6. 84000 | 3. 30000 | 10. 90000 | 1. 70000 |
| 7. 20000 | 3. 40000 | 11. 10000 | 1. 80000 |
| 7. 56000 | 3. 50000 | 11. 20000 | 1. 90000 |
| 7. 92000 | 3. 60000 | 11. 30000 | 2. 05000 |
| 8. 28000 | 3. 70000 | 11. 40000 | 2. 15000 |
| 8. 64000 | 3. 80000 | 11. 50000 | 2. 30000 |
| 9. 00000 | 3. 90000 | 11. 60000 | 2. 45000 |
| 9. 36000 | 3. 90000 | 11. 70000 | 2. 60000 |
| 9. 72000 | 4. 00000 | 11. 80000 | 2. 65000 |
| 10. 08000 | 4. 10000 | 11. 90000 | 2. 80000 |
| 10. 44000 | 4. 20000 | | 2. 90000 |
| 10. 80000 | 4. 20000 | | 2. 95000 |

S 5

| Flexion moment [Nm] | Angular deformity | | Internal fixator [degrees] |
|---|---|---|---|
| | intact spine [degrees] | lesion [degrees] | |
| 11. 52000 | 4. 40000 | | 3. 20000 |
| 12. 24000 | 4. 40000 | | 3. 80000 |
| 12. 96000 | 4. 40000 | | 4. 10000 |
| 13. 68000 | 4. 50000 | | 4. 40000 |
| 14. 40000 | 4. 60000 | | 4. 80000 |
| 15. 12000 | 4. 60000 | | 5. 30000 |
| 15. 84000 | 4. 70000 | | 5. 90000 |
| 16. 56000 | 4. 70000 | | 6. 20000 |
| 17. 28000 | 4. 80000 | | 6. 60000 |
| 18. 00000 | 4. 80000 | | 7. 00000 |
| 18. 71999 | 4. 90000 | | 7. 40000 |
| 19. 43999 | 5. 00000 | | 7. 80000 |
| 20. 15999 | 5. 00000 | | 8. 20000 |
| 20. 87999 | | | 8. 60000 |
| 21. 59999 | | | 9. 00000 |

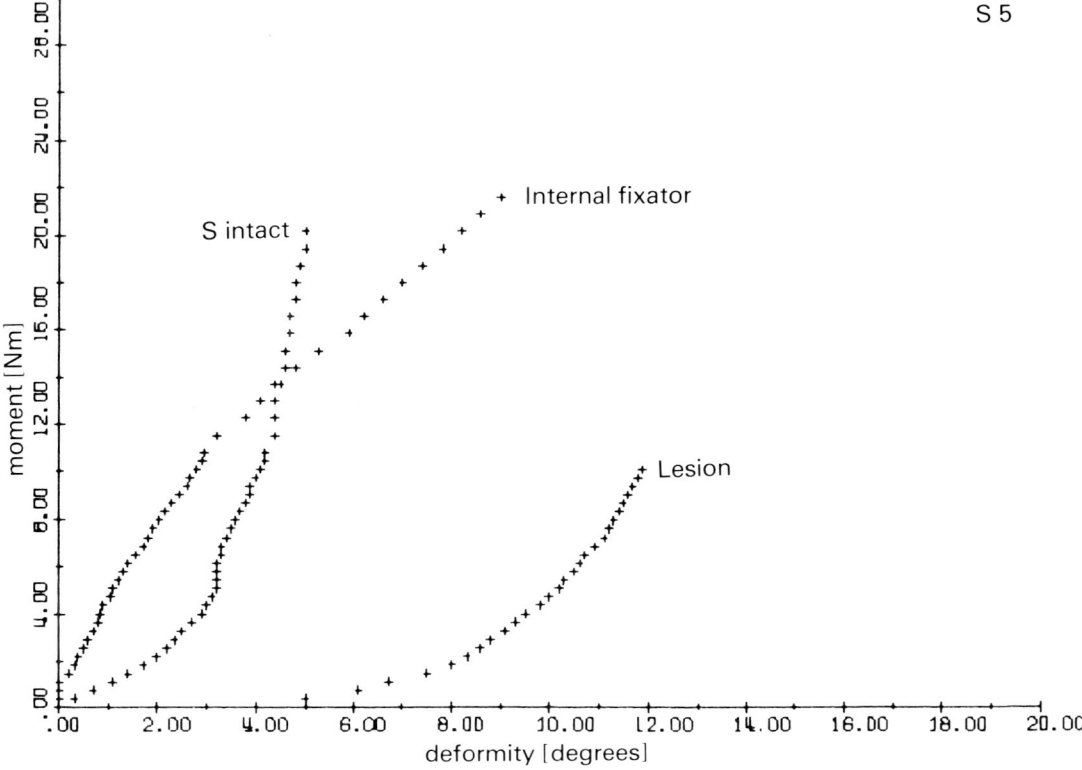

Fig. 123. Specimen S 5

Spine 6: no. 367/83; female, 78 years old.

Table 14. Specimen S6

S 6

| Flexion moment [Nm] | Angular deformity intact spine [degrees] | lesion [degrees] | Internal fixator [degrees] |
|---|---|---|---|
| .36000 | .30000 | 3.50000 | .00000 |
| .72000 | .60000 | 5.70000 | .30000 |
| 1.08000 | 1.00000 | 11.90000 | .60000 |
| 1.44000 | 1.30000 | 12.40000 | .70000 |
| 1.80000 | 1.50000 | 13.00000 | .75000 |
| 2.16000 | 1.70000 | 13.90000 | .80000 |
| 2.52000 | 1.70000 | 14.30000 | .80000 |
| 2.88000 | 1.70000 | | .80000 |
| 3.24000 | 1.80000 | | .80000 |
| 3.60000 | 1.85000 | | .90000 |
| 3.96000 | 2.10000 | | .95000 |
| 4.32000 | 2.20000 | | 1.00000 |
| 4.68000 | 2.40000 | | 1.00000 |
| 5.04000 | 2.50000 | | 1.00000 |
| 5.40000 | 2.70000 | | 1.00000 |
| 5.76000 | 2.90000 | | 1.00000 |
| 6.12000 | 3.10000 | | 1.05000 |
| 6.48000 | 3.20000 | | 1.20000 |
| 6.84000 | 3.30000 | | 1.35000 |
| 7.20000 | 3.40000 | | 1.50000 |
| 7.56000 | 3.50000 | | 1.60000 |
| 7.92000 | 3.70000 | | 1.65000 |
| 8.28000 | 3.80000 | | 1.80000 |
| 8.64000 | 3.80000 | | 1.90000 |
| 9.00000 | 3.90000 | | 2.00000 |
| 9.36000 | 4.05000 | | 2.10000 |
| 9.72000 | 4.25000 | | 2.30000 |
| 10.08000 | 4.40000 | | 2.40000 |
| 10.44000 | 4.70000 | | 2.60000 |

S 6

| Flexion moment [Nm] | Angular deformity intact spine [degrees] | lesion [degrees] | Internal fixator [degrees] |
|---|---|---|---|
| 10.80000 | 4.70000 | | 2.90000 |
| 11.52000 | 4.90000 | | 3.30000 |
| 12.24000 | 5.10000 | | 4.00000 |
| 12.96000 | 5.10000 | | 4.50000 |
| 13.68000 | 5.30000 | | 5.10000 |
| 14.40000 | 5.50000 | | 6.00000 |
| 15.12000 | 5.70000 | | 6.60000 |
| 15.84000 | 5.80000 | | 7.30000 |
| 16.56000 | | | 8.20000 |
| 17.28000 | | | 8.90000 |
| 18.00000 | | | 9.70000 |
| 18.71999 | | | 10.60000 |
| 19.43999 | | | 11.40000 |

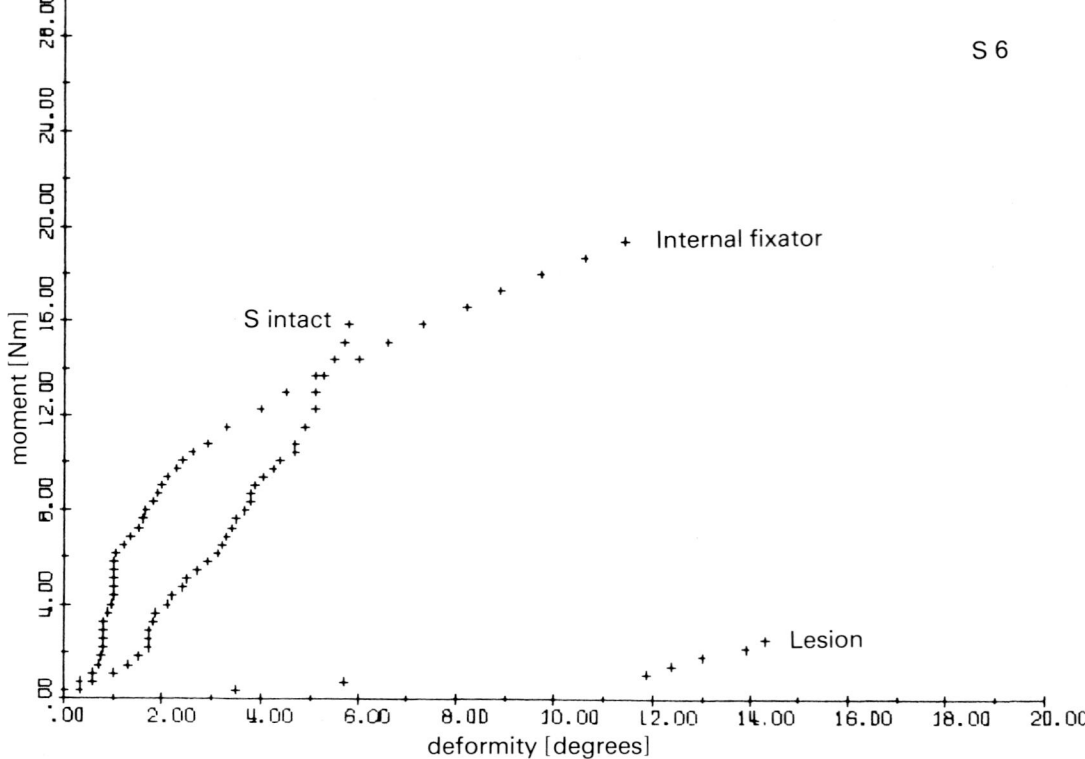

Fig. 124. Specimen S6

## Spine 7: no. 421/83; female, 79 years old.

Table 15. Specimen S7

S 7

| Flexion moment [Nm] | Angular deformity intact spine [degrees] | lesion [degrees] | Internal fixator [degrees] |
|---|---|---|---|
| .36000 | .30000 | 2.00000 | .05000 |
| .72000 | .50000 | 3.00000 | .05000 |
| 1.08000 | .80000 | 6.20000 | .05000 |
| 1.44000 | 1.20000 | 7.70000 | .10000 |
| 1.80000 | 1.50000 | 8.40000 | .10000 |
| 2.16000 | 1.70000 | 9.60000 | .20000 |
| 2.52000 | 1.90000 | 10.40000 | .25000 |
| 2.88000 | 2.10000 | 10.90000 | .35000 |
| 3.24000 | 2.30000 | 11.20000 | .45000 |
| 3.60000 | 2.40000 | 11.60000 | .55000 |
| 3.96000 | 2.50000 | 12.10000 | .60000 |
| 4.32000 | 2.70000 | 12.60000 | .70000 |
| 4.68000 | 2.80000 | 13.00000 | .85000 |
| 5.04000 | 3.00000 | 13.50000 | .90000 |
| 5.40000 | 3.20000 | 13.90000 | 1.00000 |
| 5.76000 | 3.30000 | 14.60000 | 1.05000 |
| 6.12000 | 3.40000 | | 1.20000 |
| 6.48000 | 3.60000 | | 1.30000 |
| 6.84000 | 3.80000 | | 1.40000 |
| 7.20000 | 3.90000 | | 1.50000 |
| 7.56000 | 4.10000 | | 1.70000 |
| 7.92000 | 4.20000 | | 1.90000 |
| 8.64000 | 4.50000 | | 2.10000 |
| 9.36000 | 4.70000 | | 2.50000 |
| 10.08000 | 5.00000 | | 2.80000 |
| 10.80000 | 5.20000 | | 3.10000 |
| 11.52000 | 5.40000 | | 3.50000 |
| 12.24000 | 5.50000 | | 4.10000 |
| 12.96000 | 5.70000 | | 4.70000 |

S 7

| Flexion moment [Nm] | Angular deformity intact spine [degrees] | lesion [degrees] | Internal fixator [degrees] |
|---|---|---|---|
| 13.68000 | 5.90000 | | 5.50000 |
| 14.40000 | 6.10000 | | 6.30000 |
| 15.12000 | 6.30000 | | 7.00000 |
| 15.84000 | 6.50000 | | 7.60000 |
| 16.56000 | 6.70000 | | 8.50000 |
| 17.28000 | 6.90000 | | 9.50000 |
| 18.00000 | 7.10000 | | 10.30000 |
| 18.71999 | 7.30000 | | 11.00000 |

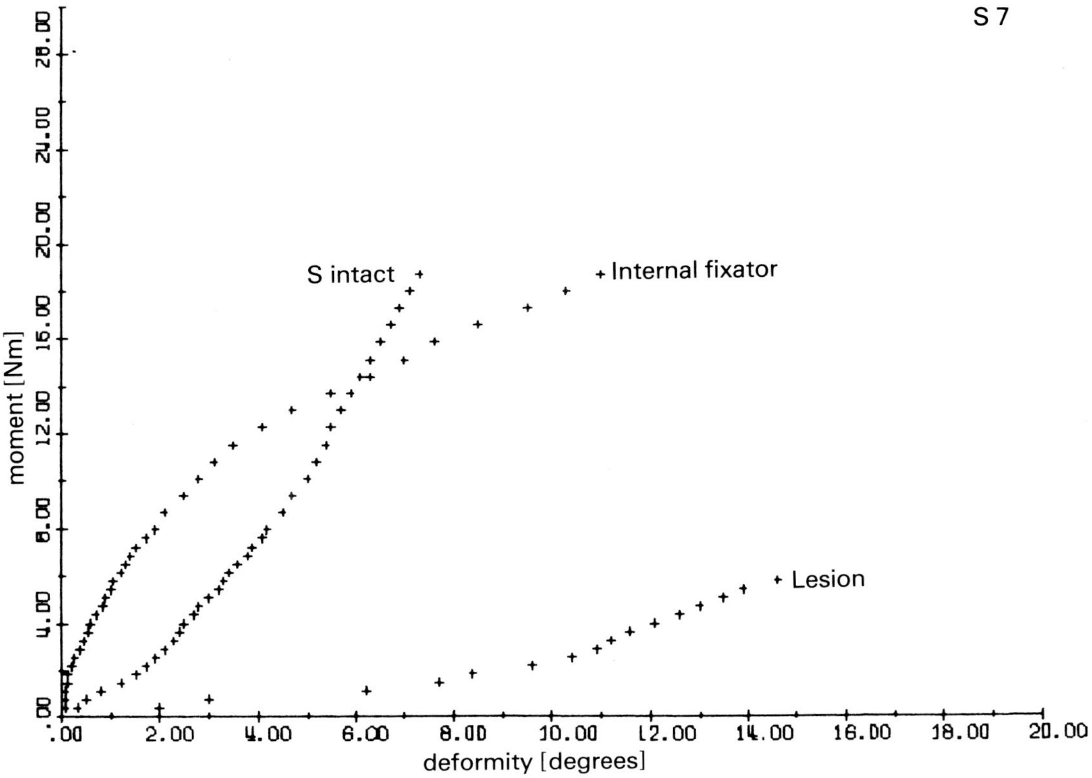

Fig. 125. Specimen S7

# 12. References

1  AEBI, M., MOHLER, J., ZÄCH, G.A., MORSCHER, E. (1983): Die operative Behandlung von Halswirbelsäulenverletzungen. Helv. chir. Acta 50, 199.

2  AKBARNIA, B.A., FOGARTY, J.P., TAYOB, A.A. (1984): Contoured Harrington instrumentation in the treatment of unstable spinal fractures. The effect of supplementary sublaminar wires. Clin. Orthop. 189, 186–194.

3  ALBEE, F.H. (1911): Transplantation of a portion of the tibia into the spine for Pott's disease. JAMA 57, 885.

4  ANDÉN, U., LAKE, A., NORDWALL, A. (1980): The role of the anterior longitudinal ligament in Harrington rod fixation of unstable thoracolumbar spinal fractures. Spine 5, 23.

5  ANDERSON, L.D., SMITH, B.L., DE TORRE, J., LITTLETON, J.T. (1982): The role of polytomography in the diagnosis and treatment of cervical spine injuries. Clin. Orthop. 165, 64.

6  ARMSTRONG, G.W.D., JOHNSTON, D.H. (1974): Stabilization of spinal injuries using Harrington instrumentation. J. Bone. Jt. Surg. 56B, 590.

7  ARNOLD, W. (1985): Operative Frühbehandlung mit dem Fixateur externe bei traumatischer Querschnittslähmung. Beitr. Orthop. Traumatol. 32, 6–14.

8  BAILEY, R.W., BADGLEY, C.E. (1960): Stabilization of the cervical spine by anterior fusion. J. Bone Jt. Surg. 42A, 565.

9  BEDBROOK, G.M. (1979): Spinal injuries with tetraplegia and paraplegia. J. Bone Jt. Surg. 61B, 267.

10  BLAIMONT, P., ALAMEH, M. (1981): Biomécanique de l'arthrodèse lombaire. Acta Orthop. Belgica 47, 605.

11  BÖHLER, J. (1981): Schraubenosteosynthese von Frakturen des Dens Axis. Unfallheilkunde 84, 221.

12  BÖHLER, J. (1982): Anterior stabilization for acute fractures and non-unions of the dens. J. Bone Jt. Surg. 64A, 18.

13  BÖHLER, J., GAUDERNAK, T. (1980): Anterior plate stabilization for fracture-dislocations of the lower cervical spine. J. Trauma 20, 203.

14  BÖHLER, L. (1932): Die Behandlung der Wirbelbrüche. Arch. klin. Chir. 173, 842.

15  BÖTEL, U. (1979): Stabilisierung und Frühmobilisation bei Verrenkungsbrüchen der Rumpfwirbelsäule mit der Weiss-Feder. Unfallheilkunde 82, 108.

16  BÖTEL, U. (1980): Die Behandlung der Verrenkungs-

brüche der Brust- und Lendenwirbelsäule mit der Weiss-Feder und ihre Modifikationen. Hefte z. Unfallheilkunde *149*, 182.

17  BOHLMAN, H.H. (1974): Traumatic fractures of the upper thoracic spine with paralysis. J. Bone Jt. Surg. *56A*, 1299.

18  BOHLMAN, H.H., EISMONT, F.J. (1981): Surgical techniques of anterior decompression and fusion for spinal cord injuries. Clin. Orthop. *154*, 57.

19  BOHLMAN, H.H., COOK, S.S. (1982): One-stage decompression and posterolateral and interbody fusion for lumbosacral spondyloptosis through a posterior approach. J. Bone Jt. Surg. *64A*, 415–418.

20  BOHLMAN, H.H. (1985): Treatment of fractures and dislocations of the thoracic and lumbar spine. J. Bone Jt. Surg. *67A*, 165–169.

21  BOIJSEN, E., EKELUND, L. (1983): Computed tomography in orthopedic trauma. In: Boijsen, E., Ekelund, F. (Eds.): Computed tomography in orthopedic radiology. Thieme, Stuttgart/New York.

22  BOLAND, P.J., LANE, J.M., SUNDARESAN, N. (1982): Metastatic disease of the spine. Clin. Orthop. *169*, 95.

23  BOSWORTH, D.M. (1942): Clothespine or inclusion graft for spondylolisthesis or laminal defects of the lumbar spine. Surgery, Gynecology and Obstetrics *75*, 593.

24  BOXALL, D., BRADFORD, D.S., WINTER, R.B., MOE, J.H. (1979): Management of severe spondylolisthesis in children and adolescents. J. Bone Jt. Surg. *61A*, 479–495.

25  BRADFORD, D.S., AKBARNIA, B.A., WINTER, B., SELJESKOG, E.L. (1977): Surgical stabilization of fracture dislocations of the thoracic spine. Spine *2*, 185.

26  CASPAR, W. (1982): A new metal plate for stabilization of unstable fractures dislocations of the cervical spine. In: International college of surgeons, austrian section, I. Viennese workshop, Vienna, October 3–6, 1982: p.88.

27  CLARK, W.K.(1981): Spinal cord decompression in spinal cord injury. Clin. Orthop. *154*, 9.

28  CLOWARD, R.B. (1961): Treatment of acute fractures and fracture-dislocations of the cervical spine by vertebral body fusion. J. Neurosurg. *18*, 201.

29  CONVERY, F.R., MINTEER, M.A., SMITH, R.W., EMERSON, S.M. (1978): Fracture-dislocation of the dorsolumbar spine. Acute operative stabilization by Harrington instrumentation. Spine *3*, 160.

30  COMARR, A.E., KAUFMAN, A.A. (1956): A survey of the neurological results of 858 spinal cord injuries: a comparison of patients treated with and without laminectomy. J. Neurosurg. *13*, 95–106.

31  DANIAUX, H. (1986): Transpedikuläre Reposition und Spongiosaplastik bei Wirbelkörperbrüchen der unteren Brust- und Lendenwirbelsäule. Unfallchirurgie *89*, 197–213.

32  DANIAUX, H. (1982): Technik und erste Ergebnisse der transpedikulären Spongiosaplastik bei Kompressionsbrüchen im Lendenwirbelsäulenbereich. Acta Chir. Austriaca, Supplement *43*, 79.

33  DAVIES, W.E., MORRIS, J.H., HILL, V. (1980): An analysis of conservative (non-surgical) management of thoracolumbar fractures and fracture-dislocations with neural damage. J. Bone Jt. Surg. *62A*, 1324.

34  DAVIES, W.E. (1981): Reply to the letter to the editor of R.R.Jacobs and M.A.Asher. J. Bone Jt. Surg. *63A*, 1033.

35  DENIS, F. (1984): Spinal instability defined by the three-column spine concept in acute spinal trauma. Clin. Orthop. *189*, 65–76.

36  DEWALD, R.L., FAUT, M.M., TADDONIO, R.F., NEUWIRTH, M.G. (1981): Severe lumbo-sacral spondylolisthesis in adolescents and children. J. Bone Jt. Surg. *63A*, 619–626.

37  DICK, W. (1983): Die Indikation zur Osteosynthese von Wirbelfrakturen. In: Morscher, E., Harder, F., Rutishauser, G., Frede, F.E. (Hrsg.): Entwicklungen in der Chirurgie. Schwabe, Basel.

38  DICK, W., MORSCHER, E., ZÄCH, G. (1982): Differential-Indikation zur operativen Frühbehandlung von Wirbelsäulenverletzungen. Acta Chir. Austriaca, Supplement *43*, 67.

39  DICK, W., KLUGER, P., MAGERL, F., WÖRSDÖRFER, O., ZÄCH, G. (1985): A new device for internal fixation of thoracolumbar and lumbar spine fractures: the «Fixateur interne». Paraplegia *23*, 225–232.

40  DICK, W., (1986): Use of the acetabular reamer to harvest autogenic bone graft material: a simple method for producing bone paste. Arch. Orthop. Trauma Surg. *105*, 235–238.

41  DICK, W., MORSCHER, E. Therapiekonzept für die Spondylolisthesis. In: Hohmann, D., Kügelgen, B., Liebig, K. (Hrsg.): Neuroorthopädie 4. Springer, Heidelberg/New York/Tokyo (in press).

42  DICK, W., WÖRSDÖRFER, D., MAGERL, F. (1985): Mechanical properties of a new device for internal fixation of spine fractures: the «Fixateur interne», Vol.2. In: Perren, S.M., Schneider, E.V. (Eds.): Developments in Biomechanics, pp.501–506. Nijhoff, The Hague.

43  DICKSON, J.H., HARRINGTON, P.R., ERWIN, W.D. (1978): Results of reduction and stabilization of the severely fractured thoracic and lumbar spine. J. Bone Jt. Surg. *60A*, 799.

44  DOLANC, B. (1980): Operative Behandlung bei Frakturen Th11–L5. Hefte z. Unfallheilkunde *149*, 169.

45  DUNN, H.K. (1984): Anterior stabilization of thorakolumbar injuries. Clin. Orthop. *189*, 116–124.

46  DURWARD, Q.J., SCHWEIGEL, J.F., HARRISON, PH. (1981): Management of fractures of the thoracolumbar and lumbar spine. Neurosurgery *8*, 555.

47  DWYER, A.F. (1974): Experience of anterior approach to scoliosis. Results of treatment in 51 cases. J. Bone Jt. Surg. *56B*, 218.

48  FERGUSON, R.L. (1983): The evolution of segmental spinal instrumentation in the treatment of unstable thoracolumbar spine fractures. J. Pediatr. Orthop. *3*, 124.

49  FLESH, J.R., LEIDER, L.L., ERICKSON, D.L., CHOU, S.N., BRADFORD, D.S. (1977): Harrington instrumentation and spine fusion for unstable fractures and fracture-dislocations of the thoracic and lumbar spine. J. Bone Jt. Surg. *59A*, 143.

50  FRANKEL, H.L., HANCOCK, D.O., HYSLOP, G., MEL-

ZAK, J., MICHAELIS, L.S., UNGAR, G.H., VERNON, J.D.S., WALSH, J.J. (1969): The value of postural reduction in the initial mangement of closed injuries of the spine with paraplegia and tetraplegia. Paraplegia 7, 179.

51 FREDERICKSON, B.E., BAKER, D., MCHOLICK, W.J., YUAN, H.A., LUBICKY, J.P. (1984): The natural history of spondylolysis and spondylolisthesis. J. Bone Jt. Surg. 66A, 699–707.

52 GAINES et al. (1983): Harrington distraction rods supplemented with sublaminar wires for thoracolumbar fracture dislocation – experimental and clinical investigation. In: Meeting highlights. J. Pediatr. Orthop. 3, 124.

53 GAINES, R.W., BREEDLOVE, R.F., MUNSON, G. (1984): Stabilization of thoracic and thoracolumbar fracture-dislocations with Harrington rods and sublaminar wires. Clin. Orthop. 189, 195–203.

54 GERTZBEIN, S.D., MACMICHAEL, D., TILE, M. (1982): Harrington instrumentation as a method of fixation in fractures of the spine. A critical analysis of deficiencies. J. Bone Jt. Surg. 64B, 526.

55 GLENN, W.V., RHODES, M.L., ALTSCHULER, L.L., WILTSE, C., KOSTANEK, C., MING KUO, Y. (1979): Multiplanar display computerized bony tomography applications in the lumbar spine. Spine 4, 282.

56 GREEN, B.A., CALLAHAN, R.A., KLOSE, K.J., DE LA TORRE, J. (1981): Acute spinal cord injury: Current concepts. Clin. Orthop. 154, 125.

57 GRISS, P., JANI, L. (1983): Die Kombination Harrington-Luque, biomechanisches Prinzip und erste klinische Ergebnisse. Vortrag V. Münchner Symposion für experimentelle Orthopädie, 11.–12.2.1983.

58 GROTE, W., ROOSEN, C. (1981): Indikationen und Technik der zervikalen ventralen Wirbelkörperfusion mit Knochenzement. Z. Orthop. 119, 728.

59 GRUCA, A. (1956): Protocol for the 41st Congress of Indian Orthopaedics and Traumatology, Bologna. Zit. nach: White, A.A., Panjabi, M.M., Thomas, C.L. (1977).

60 GRUCA, A. (1960): Muscle alloplasty in scoliosis. Chirurg. Narz. Ruchi i Ortoped. 2, 167 (zit. nach Weiss, M.).

61 GUMLEY, G., TAYLOR, T.K.F., RYAN, M.D. (1982): Distraction fractures of the lumbar spine. J. Bone Jt. Surg. 64B, 520.

62 GUTTMANN, L. (1949) Surgical aspects of the treatment of traumatic paraplegia. J. Bone. Jt. Surg. 31B, 399.

63 GUTTMANN, L. (1969): Die initiale Behandlung von Querschnittslähmungen des Rückenmarkes nach Frakturen der Wirbelsäule. Die Wirbelsäule in Forschung und Praxis 42, 58

64 HADRA, B.E. (1891): Wiring of the vertebrae as a means of immobilization in fracture and Pott's disease. Medical Times and Register 22, 423. Reprint: Clin. Orthop. 112, (1975).

65 HALL, A.J., MACKAY, N.N. (1973): The results of laminectomy for compression of the cord or cauda equina by extradural malignant tumor. J. Bone Jt. Surg. 55B, 497.

66 HARMS, J., STOLTZE, D., GRASS, M. (1985): Operative Behandlung der Spondylolisthesis durch dorsale Reposition und ventrale Fusion. Orthop. Praxis 12, 996–1001.

67 HARRINGTON, K.D. (1981): The use of methylmethacrylate for vertebral body replacement and anterior stabilization of pathological fracture-dislocations of the spine due to metastatic disease. J. Bone Jt. Surg. 63A, 36.

68 HARRINGTON, P.R. (1962): Treatment of scoliosis. Correction and internal fixation by spine instrumentation. J. Bone Jt. Surg. 44A, 591.

69 HARRINGTON, P.R. (1967): Instrumentation in spine instability other than scoliosis. S. Afr. J. Surg. 5, 7.

70 HARRINGTON, P.R. (1972): Technical details in relationship to the successful use of instrumentation in scoliosis. Orthop. Clinics North Amer. 3, 49.

71 HARRINGTON, P.R., DICKSON, J.H. (1973): The development and further prospects of internal fixation of the spine. Israel J. Med. Sci. 9, 773.

72 HARRINGTON, P.R., DICKSON, J.H. (1976): Spinal instrumentation in the treatment of severe progressive spondylolisthesis. Clin. Orthop. 117, 157–163.

73 HASDAY, C.A., PASSOFF, T.L., PERRY, J. (1983): Gait abnormalities from iatrogenic loss of lumbar lordosis secondary to Harrington lumbar fractures. Spine 8, 501.

73a HEFTI, F., DICK, W. (1986): PDS-Posterior derotation system; a new operative technique for the treatment of thoracolumbar and lumbar scoliosis. European Deformities Society First Congress «Scoliosis: the last 20 years experience», Rome, April 16–19, 1986, Abstract book.

74 HERRING, J.A., WENGER, D.R. (1982): Segmental spinal instrumentation. A preliminary report of 40 consecutive cases. Spine 7, 282.

75 HIBBS, R.A. (1911): An operation for progressive spinal deformities. N.Y. Med. J. 93, 1013.

76 HOLDSWORTH, F.W., HARDY, A. (1953): Early treatment of paraplegia from fractures of the thoraco-lumbar spine. J. Bone Jt. Surg. 35B, 540.

77 HOLDSWORTH, F. (1963): Fractures, dislocations, and fracture-dislocations of the spine. J. Bone Jt. Surg. 45B, 6.

78 HOLDSWORTH, F. (1970): Fractures, dislocations, and fracture-dislocations of the spine. J. Bone Jt. Surg. 52A, 1534.

79 HOLM, ST., NACHEMSON, A. (1982): Nutritional changes in the canine intervertebral disc after spinal fusion. Clin. Orthop. 169, 243.

80 HOPF, A. (1958): Die Verletzungen der Wirbelsäule. In: Hohmann, G., Hackenbroch, M., Lindemann, K. (Hrsg.): Handbuch der Orthopädie, Band II, S.458–536. Thieme, Stuttgart.

81 JACOBS, R.R., ASHER, M.A., SNIDER, R.K. (1980): Dorso-lumbale Wirbelsäulenfrakturen – eine vergleichende Studie zwischen konservativer und operativer Behandlung bei 100 Patienten. Orthopäde 9, 45.

82 JACOBS, R.R., DAHNERS, L.E., GERTZBEIN, S.D., NORDWALL, A., MATHYS, R. (1983): A locking hook-spinal rod: current status of development. Paraplegia 21, 197–200.

83 JACOBS, R.R., NORDWALL, A., NACHEMSON, A.L. (1982): Reduction, stability, and strength provided by internal fixation systems for thoracolumbar spinal injuries. Clin. Orthop. *171*, 300–308.

84 JACOBS, R.R., SCHLAEPFER, F., MATHYS, R., NACHEMSON, A., PERREN, S.M. (1979): A locking hook spinal rod system for fracture-dislocations of the dorso-lumbar spine: a biomechanical evaluation. Vortrag European Society of Biomechanics, Strasbourg, France, September 14, 1979.

85 JACOBS, R.R., SCHLAEPFER, F., MATHYS, R., PERREN, S.M. (1980): An experimental spinal instrumentation system for traumatic instability of the dorso-lumbar spine. J. Biomech. *13*, 801.

86 JACOBS, R.R., CASEY, M. (1984): Surgical management of thoracolumbar spinal injuries. Clin. Orthop. *189*, 22–35.

87 JAFFE, W.L. (1958): Tumors and tumorous conditions of the bones and joints. Lea & Febinger, Philadelphia.

88 JUNGHANNS, H. (1973): Metallfixation von Knochenblocks an der Halswirbelsäule. Chirurg *44*, 87.

89 KAHANOWITZ, N., ARNOCZKY, S.P., LEVINE, D.B., OTIS, J.P. (1984): The effects of internal fixation on the articular cartilage of unfused canine facet joint cartilage. Spine *9*, 268–272.

90 KAHANOWITZ, N., BULLOUGH, P., JACOBS, R.R. (1984): The effect of internal fixation without arthrodesis on human facet joint cartilage. Clin. Orthop. *189*, 204–208.

91 KANEDA, K., ABUMI, K., FUJIYA, M. (1984): Burst fractures with neurologic deficits of the thoraco-lumbar spine. Results of anterior decompression and stabilization with anterior instrumentation. Spine *9*, 788–795.

92 KAUFER, H., HAYES, J.T. (1966): Lumbar fracture-dislocation. A study of twenty-one cases. J. Bone Jt. Surg. *48A*, 712.

93 KEMPF, J., ISSA, J.B., BRIOT, B., GROSSE, A., JAEGER, J.H., LEMAGUET, A., DELANGRE, C. (1980): Traitement chirurgical des fractures instables du rachis dorso-lombaire par matériel de Harrington. Acta Orthop. Belgica *46*, 289.

94 KEMPF, J., RENAULT, D., LE MAGUET, A., CLAVIER, J., JAEGER, J.H., MUSTER, D. (1980): Biomechanical study of dorso-lumbar spine osteosynthesis with reversed Harrington rods and hooks and Roy-Camille plates. Acta Orthop. Belgica *46*, 829.

95 KINZL, L. (1980): Operative Therapie der thorakalen Wirbelfrakturen. Hefte z. Unfallheilkunde *149*, 161.

96 KLUGER, P. (1983): Ein neues Zielprinzip zur axialen Ausrichtung im Röntgenstrahlengang. Chirurg *54*, 427.

97 KLUGER, G., GERNER, H.J. (1986): Das mechanische Prinzip des Fixateur externe zur dorsalen Stabilisierung der Brust- und Lendenwirbelsäule. Unfallchirurgie *12*, 68–79.

98 KORTMANN, H.: Unfallchirurg. Abt., Allgemeines Krankenhaus St.Georg, D-2000 Hamburg 1, Germany: unpublished data.

99 KOSTUIK, J.P. (1984): Anterior fixation for fractures of the thoracic and lumbar spine with or without neurologic involvments. Clin. Orthop. *189*, 103–115.

100 KRAG, M.H., BEYNNON, B.D., POPE, M.H., FRYMOYER, J.W., HAUGH, L.D., WEAVER, D.L. (1986): An internal fixator for posterior application to short segments of the thoracic, lumbar or lumbosacral spine. Design and testing. Clin. Orthop. *203*, 75–98.

101 LABORDE, M., BAHNIUK, E., BOHLMAN, H.H., SAMSON, B. (1980): Comparison of Fixation of Spinal Fractures. Clin. Orthop. *152*, 303–310.

102 LAUSBERG, G. (1969): Ist die operative Behandlung der Wirbelsäulenverletzung mit Rückenmarksbeteiligung angezeigt? Die Wirbelsäule in Forschung und Praxis *42*, 80.

103 LEWIS, J., McKIBBIN, B. (1974): The treatment of unstable fracture-dislocations of the thoraco-lumbar spine accompanied by paraplegia. J. Bone Jt. Surg. *56B*, 603.

104 LINDAHL, S., WILLEN, J., IRSTAM, L. (1983): Computed tomography of bone fragments in the spinal canal. Spine *8*, 181.

105 LOB, A. (1954): Die Wirbelsäulenverletzungen und ihre Ausheilung. Thieme, Stuttgart.

106 LOKIETEK, W. (1981): La vertébrectomie dans la rachis tumoral, inflammatoire, traumatique. Acta Orthop. Belgica *47*, 705.

107 LOUIS, R. (1982): Chirurgie du rachis. Anatomie chirurgicale et voies d'abord. Springer, Berlin/Heidelberg/New York.

108 LOUIS, R., MARESCA, C. (1977): Stabilisation chirurgicale avec réduction des spondylolysis et des spondylolisthesis. Int. Orthop. *1*, 215–225.

109 LUQUE, E. (1982): Segmental spinal instrumentation for correction of scoliosis. Clin. Orthop. *163*, 192.

110 LUQUE, E. (1982): Paralytic scoliosis in growing children. Clin. Orthop. *163*, 202.

111 LUQUE, E., CASSIS, N., RAMIREZ-WIELLA, G. (1982): Segmental spinal instrumentation in the treatment of fractures of the thoracolumbar spine. Spine *7*, 312.

112 MacNAB, J. (1977): Backache, Williams and Wilkins, Baltimore.

113 MAGERL, F. (1979): Die Behandlung von Wirbelsäulenverletzungen. In: von Wayand, E., Brücke, P. (Hrsg.): Kongressbericht 19. Tgg. Öst. Ges. f. Chirurgie, Band II, S.859. Egermann, Wien.

114 MAGERL, F. (1980): Operative Frühbehandlung bei traumatischer Querschnittlähmung. Orthopäde *9*, 34.

115 MAGERL, F. (1980): Verletzungen der Brust- und Lendenwirbelsäule. Langenbecks Arch. Chir. *352*, 427.

116 MAGERL, F. (1981): Clinical application on the thoraco-lumbar junction and the lumbar spine with a fixateur externe. In: Mears, D.C. (Ed.): External skeletal fixation. Williams and Wilkins, Baltimore.

117 MAGERL, F. (1982): External skeletal fixation of the lower thoracic and the lumbar spine. In: Uhthoff, H.K. (Ed): Current concepts of external fixation of fractures, pp.353–366. Springer, Berlin/Heidelberg/New York.

118 MAGERL, F. (1982): Spondylodesen an der oberen Halswirbelsäule. Acta Chir. Austriaca, Supplement *43*, 69.

119 MAGERL, F. (1982): Stabilisierung der unteren Brust- und der Lendenwirbelsäule mit dem Fixateur externe. Acta Chir. Austriaca, Supplement *43*, 78.

120 MAGERL, F.: Orthopedic Clinic, Kantonsspital St. Gallen (Switzerland), personal communication.

121 MAGNUS, G. (1930): Die Behandlung und Begutachtung des Wirbelbruches. Arch. orthop. Unfall-Chir. *29*, 277.

122 MALCOLM, B.W. (1979): Spinal deformity secondary to spinal injury. Orthop. Clin. North America *10*, 943.

123 MARKWALDER, H. (1966): Indikationen zur chirurgischen Behandlung von Wirbelsäulen- und Rückenmarksverletzungen im Frühstadium. In: Rehabilitation der Para- und Tetraplegiker. Fortbildungskurs 3. März 1966, Bern: Organisation Schweizerische Rehabilitationskommission.

124 MCAFEE, P.C., YUAN, H.A., FREDERICKSON, B.E., LUBICKY, J.P. (1983): The value of computed tomography in thoraco-lumbar fractures. J. Bone Jt. Surg. *65A*, 461.

125 MCAFEE, P.C., BOHLMAN, H.H. (1985): Complications following Harrington instrumentation for fractures of the thoracolumbar spine. J. Bone Jt. Surg. *67A*, 672–686.

126 MCAFEE, P.C., BOHLMAN, H.H., YUAN, H.A. (1983): Anterior decompression of traumatic thoracolumbar fractures with incomplete neurological deficit using a retroperitoneal approach. J. Bone Jt. Surg. *65A*, 461–473.

127 MOON, M.S., KIM, J., WOO, Y.K., LEE, J.J. (1981): Anterior interbody fusion in fractures and fracture-dislocations of the spine. International Orthopaedics (SICOT) *5*, 143.

128 MORGAN, T.H., WHARTON, G.W., AUSTIN, G.N. (1971): The results of laminectomy in patients with incomplete spinal cord injuries. Paraplegia *9*, 14.

129 MORSCHER, E. (1970): Operative Aufrichtung fixierter Hyperkyphosen durch vordere Wirbelsäulenosteotomie. Z. Orthop. *108*, 516.

130 MORSCHER, E. (1972): Operative Aufrichtung von Wirbelfrakturen. Mschr. Unfallheilkunde *75*, 555.

131 MORSCHER, E. (1971): Beurteilung und Behandlung von Wirbelfrakturen. Therap. Umschau *28*, 807.

132 MORSCHER, E. (1975): Zweizeitige Reposition und Stabilisation der Spondyloptose mit dem Harrington-Instrumentarium und vorderer intercorporeller Spondylodese. Arch. orthop. Unfall-Chir. *83*, 323.

133 MORSCHER, E., SUTTER, F., JENNY, H., OLERUD, S. (1986): Die vordere Verplattung der Halswirbelsäule mit dem Hohlschrauben-Plattensystem aus Titanium. Chirurg *57*, 702.

134 MORSCHER, E. (1980): Korrektur der Hyperkyphose bei frischen und alten Wirbelkompressionsfrakturen. Orthopäde *9*, 77.

135 MORSCHER, E. (1980): Klassifikation von Wirbelsäulenverletzungen. Orthopäde *9*, 2.

136 MORSCHER, E., GERBER, B., FASEL, J. (1984): Surgical treatment of spondylolisthesis by bone grafting and direct stabilization of spondylolisthesis by means of a hook screw. Arch. Orth. Trauma Surg. *103*, 175.

137 MORSCHER, E., DICK, W. (1978): Wirbelkörpereingriffe mit vorderem Zugang. Zbl. Chirurgie *103*, 1105.

138 MUHR, G., TSCHERNE, H. (1982): Die dorsale Plattenosteosynthese bei Wirbelfrakturen. Acta Chir. Austriaca, Supplement *43*, 77.

139 NACHEMSON, A.L. (1981): Disc pressure measurements. Spine *6*, 93.

140 NACHEMSON, A.L., ELFSTROM, G. (1971): Intravital wireless telemetry of axial forces in Harrington distraction rods in patients with idiopathic scoliosis. J. Bone Jt. Surg. *53A*, 445.

141 NAGEL, D.A., KOOGLE, T.A., PIZIALI, R.L., PERKASH, I.C. (1981): Stability of the upper lumbar spine following progressive disruptions and the application of individual internal and external fixation devices. J. Bone Jt. Surg. *63A*, 62.

142 NATHER, A., BOSE, K. (1982): The results of decompression of cord or cauda equina compression from metastatic extradural tumors. Clin. Orthop. *169*, 103.

143 NEUGEBAUER, J. (1981): Vergleichende Festigkeitsuntersuchungen an Wirbelsäulenimplantaten. Messtechnische Briefe *17*, 74.

144 NICOLL, E.A. (1949): Fractures of the dorso-lumbar spine. J. Bone Jt. Surg. *31B*, 376.

145 OPPEL, F., BROCK, M. (1982): Operative stabilization of the vertebral column with laminated plastic material. International college of surgeons. Austrian section. I. Viennese workshop, Vienna, October 3–6, 1982. Abstracts p. 72.

146 OPPEL, F., KUNFT, H.D. (1977): Akutversorgung von Wirbelfrakturen durch laminierte Endoprothesen: Indikation, Technik, bisherige Erfahrungen. Hefte z. Unfallheilkunde *132*, 343.

147 OROZCO DELCLOS, R., LLOVET TAPIES, J. (1970): Osteosintesis en las fractures de raquis cervical. Revista Ortop. Traumatol. *14*, 285.

148 OSEBOLD, W.R., WEINSTEIN, S.L., SPRAGUE, B.L. (1981): Thoracolumbar spine fractures: results of treatment. Spine *6*, 13.

149 PARSCH, K., PAESLACK, V. (1974): Spätfolgen der Laminektomie bei Luxationsfrakturen der Brust- und Lendenwirbelsäule mit Querschnittlähmung. Z. Orthop. *112*, 928.

150 PAUL, R.L., MICHAEL, R.H., DUNN, J.E., WILLIAMS, J.P. (1975): Anterior transthoracic surgical decompression of acute spinal cord injuries. J. Neurosurg. *43*, 299.

151 PFEIFFER, R. (1967): Fusion der Wirbelsäule mit dem Autopolymerisat Palacos. Arch. orthop. Unfall-Chir. *62*, 240.

152 POLSTER, J. (1980): Entstehungsmechanismus und Verletzungsformen von Frakturen und Luxationen. Hefte z. Unfallheilkunde *149*, 15.

153 PURCELL, G.A., MARKOLF, K.L., DAWSON, E.G. (1981): Twelfth thoracic – first lumbar vertebral mechanical stability of fractures after Harrington rod instrumentation. J. Bone Jt. Surg. *63A*, 71.

154 QUINNELL, R.C., STOCKDALE, H.R., WILLIS, D.S. (1983): Observations of pressure within normal discs in the lumbar spine. Spine *8*, 166.

155 RATHKE, F.W., SCHLEGEL, K.F. (1974): Wirbelsäule und Becken. In: Hackenbroch, M., Witt, A.N. (Hrsg): Orthopädisch-chirurgischer Operationsatlas, Bd. III. Thieme, Stuttgart.

156 RISKA, E.B. (1976): Anterolateral decompression as a treatment of paraplegia following vertebral fracture in the thoracolumbar spine. Int. Orthop. (SICOT) *1*, 22.

157 RISKA, E.B., MYLLYNEN, P. (1981): Treatment of spinal fractures with paraplegia. Zbl. Chirurgie 106, 355.

158 ROAF, R. (1960): A study of the mechanics of spinal injuries. J. Bone Jt. Surg. *42B,* 810.

159 ROBERTS, P.H. (1969): Internal metallic splintage in the treatment of traumatic paraplegia. Injury *1,* 4.

160 ROBINSON, R.A. (1959): Fusions of the cervical spine. J. Bone Jt. Surg. *41A,* 1.

161 ROBINSON, R.A. (1964): Anterior and posterior cervical spine fusions. Clin. Orthop. *35,* 34.

162 ROSENTHAL, R.E., LOWERY, E.R. (1980): Unstable fracture-dislocations of the thoracolumbar spine: results of surgical treatment. J. Trauma *20,* 485.

163 ROY-CAMILLE, R., BERTEAUX, D. (1976): Technique et résultats des ostéosynthèses du rachis lombaire par plaques postérieures vissées dans les pédicules vertébraux. Montpellier Chir. *22,* 307.

164 ROY-CAMILLE, R., SAILLANT, G., BERTEAUX, D., SALGADO, V. (1976): Osteosynthesis of thoraco-lumbar spine fractures with metal plates screwed through the vertebral pedicles. Reconstr. Surg. Traumatol. *15,* 2.

165 ROY-CAMILLE, R., SAILLANT, G., MARIE-ANNE, S., MAMOUDY, P. (1980): Behandlung von Wirbelfrakturen und -luxationen am thorako-lumbalen Übergang. Orthopäde *9,* 63.

166 ROY-CAMILLE, R., SAILLANT, G., MAZEL, C. (1986): Internal fixation of the lumbar spine with pedicle screw plating. Clin. Orthop. *203,* 7–17.

167 ROY-CAMILLE, R.: personal communication.

168 RÜTER, A., SCHULTE, J. (1980): Die Behandlung pathologischer Wirbelfrakturen. Hefte z. Unfallheilkunde *149,* 224.

169 RUGE, D. (1977): Spinal cord injuries. In: Spinal Disorders, diagnosis and treatment. Lea & Febiger, Philadelphia.

170 SAILLANT, G. (1976): Etude anatomique des pédicules vertebraux. Application chirurgicale. Rev. Chir. Orthop. *62,* 151.

171 SCHIESTEL, H. (1971): Spätschäden der Wirbelsäule nach traumatischer Gibbusbildung. Hefte z. Unfallheilkunde *108,* 87.

172 SCHLÄPFER, F., WÖRSDÖRFER, O. (1980): Methode zur Bestimmung von Kräften und Momenten im Fixateur externe, verwendet bei Instabilitäten der lumbalen Wirbelsäule. Z. Orthop. *118,* 679.

173 SCHLÄPFER, F., WÖRSDÖRFER, O., MAGERL, F., PERREN, S.M. (1982): Stabilization of the lower thoracic and lumbar spine: comparative in vitro investigation of an external skeletal and various internal fixation devices. In: Uhthoff, H.K. (Ed.): Current concepts of external fixation of fractures, p.367. Springer, Berlin/Heidelberg/New York.

174 SCHLICKE, L., SCHULAK, J. (1980): The simultaneous use of Harrington compression and distraction rods in a thoraco-lumbar fracture-dislocation. J. Trauma *20,* 177.

175 SCHÖLLNER, D. (1975): Ein neues Verfahren zur Reposition und Fixation bei Spondylolisthesis. Orthop. Praxis *11,* 270–274.

176 SCHOLL, R., DICK, W. (1983): Die operative Behandlung von Wirbelsäulentumoren. Z. Orthop. *121,* 462.

177 SCHÜRMANN, K., BUSCH, G. (1970): Die Behandlung der cervicalen Luxationsfrakturen durch die ventrale Fusion. Chirurg *41,* 225.

178 SCHWARZ, N., BÖHLER, J. (1982): Anterolaterale Dekompression und Plattenosteosynthese bei frischen Wirbelfrakturen. Acta Chir. Austriaca, Supplement *43,* 81.

179 SENEGAS, J., GAUZERE, J.M. (1976): Plaidoyer pour la chirurgie antérieure dans le traitement des traumatismes graves des cinq dernières vertèbres cervicales. Rev. Chir. Orthop. *62* (Suppl.II), 123.

180 SIJBRANDIJ, S. (1981): A new technique for the reduction and stabilization of severe spondylolisthesis. A report of two cases. J. Bone Jt. Surg. *63B,* 266–271.

181 SLOT, G.H. (1983): Correction and fixation of kyphosis with a new distraction method. Vortrag: Sommertagung 1983 der Österr. Ges. f. Orthopädie und Chirurgie, Innsbruck, 2.–4. Juni 1983.

182 SOREFF, J., AXDORPH, G., BYLUND, P., ODÉN, J., OLERUD, S. (1982): Treatment of patients with unstable fractures of the thoracic and lumbar spine. Acta orthop. scand. *53,* 369.

183 SPANUDAKIS, ST., TERBIZAN, A. (1982): Rehabilitation kompletter Querschnittgelähmter mit stabilisierten Wirbelfrakturen an der BWS und LWS. Acta Chir. Austriaca, Supplement *43,* 79.

184 SPENCE, W.T. (1973): Internal plastic splint and fusion for stabilization of the spine. Clin. Orthop. *92,* 325.

185 STAUFFER, E.S., KELLY, E.G. (1977): Fracture-dislocations of the cervical spine. J. Bone Jt. Surg. *59A,* 45.

186 STAUFFER, E.S., NEIL, J.L. (1975): Biomechanical analysis of structural stability of internal fixation in fractures of the thoracolumbar spine. Clin. Orthop. *112,* 159.

187 STAUFFER, E.S. (1984): Current concepts review: Internal fixation of fractures of the thoracolumbar spine. J. Bone Jt. Surg. *66A,* 1136–1138.

188 SUEZAWA, Y., JAKOB, H.A.C. (1986): Lumbar and Thoracic Spinal Fusion with transpedicular Fixation (Including a Novel Distraction and Compression Device). Arch. orth. Trauma Surg. *105,* 126–129.

189 SULLIVAN, J.A. et al. (1983): Management of thoracic and lumbar spine fractures with Harrington rods supplemented with segmental wires. In: Meeting highlights. J. Pediatr. Orthop. *3,* 124.

190 SZYSZKOWITZ, R., LOTTERSBERGER, E. (1982): Die Technik und Ergebnisse der hinteren Spondylodese mit Harrington-Stäben bei unstabilen Verletzungen der BWS und LWS. Acta Chir. Austriaca, Supplement *43,* 76.

191 TADMOR, R., DAVIS, K., ROBERSON, G. NEW, P., TAVERAS, J. (1978): Computed tomographic evaluation of traumatic spinal injuries. Radiology *127,* 825.

192 TESCHNER, W., MANITZ, U., HOLZWEISSIG, F., HELLINGER, J. (1983): Verankerungsversuche an menschlichen Leichenwirbelkörpern mit Hilfe von verschiedenen Schraubentypen. Z. Orthop. *121,* 206.

193 TSCHERNE, H., HIEBLER, W., MUHR, G. (1971): Zur operativen Behandlung von Frakturen und Luxationen der Halswirbelsäule. Hefte z. Unfallheilkunde *108,* 142.

194 TSCHERNE, H., MUHR, G. (1981): Technik und Ergebnisse posttraumatischer Fusionseingriffe an der Halswirbelsäule. Z. Orthop. *119,* 715.

195 ULRICH, H. (1978): Materialbelastungsprüfung bei VDS- und Dwyer-Implantaten. In: Wirbelsäule in Forschung und Praxis *72,* 116.

196 VALENCAK, E. (1979): Die vorderen operativen Zugänge zur Brust- und Lendenwirbelsäule. Acta Chir. Austriaca *6,* 121.

197 VALENCAK, E., MEZNIK, F., HORACZEK, A., VAGACS, H. (1982): Spätfolgen von Wirbelkörperfrakturen – Indikation und Ergebnisse ventraler Dekompression. Acta Chir. Austriaca, Supplement *43,* 81.

198 VELIKAS, E.P., BLACKBURNE, J.S. (1981): Surgical treatment of spondylolisthesis in children and adolescents. J. Bone Jt. Surg. *63B,* 67.

199 VERBIEST, H. (1969): Anterolateral operations for fractures and dislocations in the middle and lower parts of the cervical spine. J. Bone Jt. Surg. *51A,* 1489.

200 WANG, G.J., WHITEHILL, R., STAMP, W.G., ROSENBERGER, R. (1979): The treatment of fracture-dislocations of the thoracolumbar spine with halo-femoral traction and Harrington rod instrumentation. Clin. Orthop. *142,* 168.

201 WASYLENKO, M., SKINNER, S.R., PERRY, J., ANTONELLI, D.J. (1983): An analysis of posture and gait following spinal fusion with Harrington instrumentation. Spine *8,* 840–845.

202 WATSON-JONES, R. (1940): Fractures and other bone and joint injuries. Williams and Wilkins, Baltimore.

203 WEBER, B.G. (1966): Operative Frühbehandlung bei traumatischer Paraplegie. In: Rehabilitation der Para- und Tetraplegie. In: Rehabilitation der Para- und Tetraplegiker. Fortbildungskurs Schweiz. Rehabilitationskommission, Bern.

204 WEBER, B.G., MAGERL, F. (1978): Konservative oder operative Behandlung von Wirbelfrakturen. Helv. chir. Acta *45,* 609.

205 WEISS, M. (1975): Dynamic spine alloplasty (spring-loading corrective devices) after fracture and spinal cord injury. Clin. Orthop. *112,* 150.

206 WEISS, M., BENTKOWSKI, Z. (1974): Biomechanical study in dynamic spondylodesis of the spine. Clin. Orthop. *103,* 199.

207 WENGER, D.R., CAROLLO, J.J., WILKERSON, J.A., WAUTERS, K., HERRING, J.A. (1982): Laboratory testing of segmental spinal instrumentation versus traditional Harrington instrumentation for scoliosis treatment. Spine *7,* 265.

208 WHITE III, A.A., PANJABI, M.M. (1978): Clinical biomechanics of the spine. Lippincott, Philadelphia.

209 WHITE, A.A., PANJABI, M.M., THOMAS, C.L. (1977): The clinical biomechanics of kyphotic deformities. Clin. Orthop. *128,* 8.

210 WHITE, R.R., NEWBERG, A., SELIGSON, D (1980): Computerized tomography assessment of the traumatized dorsolumbar spine before and after Harrington instrumentation. Clin. Orthop. *146,* 150.

211 WHITESIDES, T.E., SHAH, S.G.A. (1976): On the management of unstable fractures of the thoracolumbar spine: rationale for use of anterior decompression and fusion and posterior stabilization. Spine *1,* 39.

212 WILLIAMS, E.W.M. (1963): Traumatic paraplegia. In: Matthews, D.N. (Ed.): Recent advances in the surgery of trauma, pp. 171–186. Churchill Ltd., London.

213 WILTSE, L.L., WINTER, R.B. (1983): Terminology and measurement of spondylolisthesis. J. Bone Jt. Surg. *65A,* 768–772.

214 WÖRSDÖRFER, O. (1981): Operative Stabilisierung der thorako-lumbalen und lumbalen Wirbelsäule: vergleichende biomechanische Untersuchungen zur Stabilität und Steifigkeit verschiedener dorsaler Fixationssysteme. Habilitationsschrift Klinisch-Medizinische Fakultät Ulm.

215 WÖRSDÖRFER, O., MAGERL, F. (1980): Funktionelle Anatomie der Wirbelsäule. Hefte z. Unfallheilkunde *149,* 1.

216 WÖRSDÖRFER, O.: unpublished data.

217 YOSIPOVITCH, Z., ROBIN, G.C., MAKIN, M. (1977): Open reduction of unstable thoracolumbar spine injuries and fixation with Harrington rods. J. Bone Jt. Surg. *59A,* 1003.

218 YOUNG, B., BROOKS, W.H., TIBBS, P.A. (1981): Anterior decompression and fusion for thoracolumbar fractures with neurological deficits. Acta Neurochir. *57,* 287.

219 ZÄCH, G.: Schweiz. Paraplegikerzentrum, CH–4000 Basel (Switzerland): unpublished data.

220 ZIELKE, K. (1982): Ventrale Derotationsspondylodese. Behandlungsergebnisse bei idiopathischen Lumbalskoliosen. Z. Orthop. *120,* 320.

221 ZIELKE, K., BERTHET, A. (1978): VDS – Ventrale Derotationsspondylodese. Beitr. Orthop. Traumatol. *25,* 85.

222 ZIELKE, K., PELLIN, B. (1974): Modifikation des Sakralstabes der Harrington-Implantation zur lumbosakralen Spondylodese. Arch. Orth. Unfall-Chir. *80,* 63.

223 ZIPPEL, H. (1980): Die Spondylolisthesen. Med. u. Sport *20,* 65.

The author is indebted to F. FREULER for the drawings in Fig. 44 and to B. GERBER for the drawings in Fig. 66.